Second Edition

Facilitator Guide

Self-Care for New and Student Nurses

Dorrie K. Fontaine, PhD, RN, FAAN

Tim Cunningham, DrPH, MSN, RN, FAAN

Natalie May, PhD

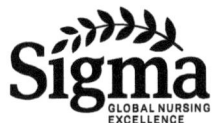

Copyright © 2025 by Sigma Theta Tau International Honor Society of Nursing

All rights reserved. This book is protected by copyright. No part of it may be reproduced, stored in a retrieval system, or transmitted in any form or by any means, electronic, mechanical, photocopying, recording, or otherwise, without written permission from the publisher. Any trademarks, service marks, design rights, or similar rights that are mentioned, used, or cited in this book are the property of their respective owners. Their use here does not imply that you may use them for a similar or any other purpose.

This book is not intended to be a substitute for the medical advice of a licensed medical professional. The author and publisher have made every effort to ensure the accuracy of the information contained within at the time of its publication and shall have no liability or responsibility to any person or entity regarding any loss or damage incurred, or alleged to have incurred, directly or indirectly, by the information contained in this book. The author and publisher make no warranties, express or implied, with respect to its content, and no warranties may be created or extended by sales representatives or written sales materials. The author and publisher have no responsibility for the consistency or accuracy of URLs and content of third-party websites referenced in this book.

Sigma Theta Tau International Honor Society of Nursing (Sigma) is a nonprofit organization whose mission is developing nurse leaders anywhere to improve healthcare everywhere. Founded in 1922, Sigma has more than 135,000 active members in over 100 countries and territories. Members include practicing nurses, instructors, researchers, policymakers, entrepreneurs, and others. Sigma's more than 540 chapters are located at more than 700 institutions of higher education throughout Armenia, Australia, Botswana, Brazil, Canada, Chile, Colombia, Croatia, England, Eswatini, Finland, Ghana, Hong Kong, Ireland, Israel, Italy, Jamaica, Japan, Jordan, Kenya, Lebanon, Malawi, Mexico, the Netherlands, Nigeria, Pakistan, Philippines, Portugal, Puerto Rico, Scotland, Singapore, South Africa, South Korea, Sweden, Taiwan, Tanzania, Thailand, the United States, and Wales. Learn more at www.sigmanursing.org.

Sigma Theta Tau International
550 West North Street
Indianapolis, IN, USA 46202

To request a review copy for course adoption, order additional books, buy in bulk, or purchase for corporate use, contact Sigma Marketplace at 888.654.4968 (US/Canada toll-free), +1.317.687.2256 (International), or solutions@sigmamarketplace.org.

To request author information, or for speaker or other media requests, contact Sigma Marketing at 888.634.7575 (US/Canada toll-free) or +1.317.634.8171 (International).

ISBN: 9781646482849
EPUB ISBN: 9781646482856
PDF ISBN: 9781646482863

Publisher: Dustin Sullivan
Acquisitions Editor: Emily Hatch
Development Editor: Jillmarie Leeper Sycamore
Cover Designer: Rebecca Batchelor
Interior Design/Page Layout: Rebecca Batchelor

Managing Editor: Carla Hall
Publications Specialist: Todd Lothery
Project Editor: Todd Lothery
Copy Editor: Erin Geile
Proofreader: Todd Lothery

About the Authors

Dorrie K. Fontaine, PhD, RN, FAAN, is the Dean Emerita at the University of Virginia (UVA) School of Nursing, where she served as Dean for 11 years until 2019. A champion of creating healthy work environments in clinical and academic settings, she is a past President of the American Association of Critical-Care Nurses (AACN). In 2009 she created the Compassionate Care Initiative at UVA, which has grown to be a guiding force in transforming the culture of the school with a focus on fostering human flourishing and resilience for students, faculty, and staff. A noted author of critical care texts, a leadership book, and multiple papers and presentations on creating healthy work environments through compassionate care, Fontaine credits a retreat at Upaya Zen Center in Santa Fe, New Mexico, with the Abbot, Roshi Joan Halifax, for setting her on the path of mindfulness, meditation, and a renewed focus on self-care. She attended Villanova University and the University of Maryland and received her PhD from The Catholic University of America. Her four-decade career of teaching and academic leadership includes the University of Maryland, Georgetown University, and the University of California, San Francisco. Working as a consultant with the Bedford Falls Foundation, she is now able to work with philanthropists who believe nurses are the future of healthcare. Fontaine lives in Charlottesville, Virginia, with her husband, Barry.

Tim Cunningham, DrPH, MSN, RN, FAAN, began his professional career as a performing artist and clown. He worked for two organizations that changed his life. The first, the Big Apple Circus, employed him to perform as a clown doctor at Boston Children's Hospital, Yale New Haven Children's Hospital, and Hasbro Children's Hospital. Concurrently, he volunteered for Clowns Without Borders (CWB), performing in various refugee camps, war zones, and other global zones of crisis. At the time of this publication, Tim is serving as Interim Executive Director of CWB. It was in pediatric hospitals and refugee camps where he witnessed and began to learn about the true meaning of resilience and self-care. The arts inspired him to pursue a career in nursing. He completed a second-degree nursing program at UVA and then became an emergency trauma nurse working clinically in Charlottesville, Virginia; Washington, DC; and New York City. It was during his time in New York that he completed his doctoral degree in public health at the Mailman School of Public Health at Columbia University. Cunningham is the former Director of the Compassionate Care Initiative at UVA, where he had the opportunity to work closely with Drs. Fontaine and May as the first edition of this book came to fruition. He currently lives in Atlanta, Georgia, where he established Emory Healthcare's Inaugural Office of Well-Being. While employed at Emory, he was Vice President, Co-Chief Well-Being Officer, and he also held a joint appointment as an Adjunct Associate Professor at the Nell Hodgson Woodruff School of Nursing at Emory University. Cunningham began his academic journey receiving his BA in English from the College of William and Mary in 2000. For self-care, Cunningham is an avid runner and wanna-be gardener. He loves any chance he can get to swim in the ocean or sit quietly as the sun rises.

Natalie May, PhD, transitioned to the UVA School of Nursing after 30 years as Associate Professor of Research in the Division of General Medicine in the UVA School of Medicine. She is a founding member of the UVA Center for Appreciative Practice. Certified as an Appreciative Inquiry facilitator and lead author of *Appreciative Inquiry in Healthcare,* she enjoys developing Appreciative Inquiry projects and teaching appreciative practice workshops at her home institution and beyond. She is an experienced qualitative researcher, and she has extensive experience in grant writing, program and curriculum development, and program evaluation. Her current research projects include the Mattering in Medicine study and the Mattering in Healthcare Education study. She was also an investigator for the Wisdom in Medicine Project: Mapping the Path Through Adversity to Wisdom, a study funded by the John Templeton Foundation. She is co-author of *Choosing Wisdom: The Path Through Adversity* and co-producer of a PBS film, *Choosing Wisdom*. She has co-developed and implemented an innovative curriculum for medical students, the Phronesis Project, designed to foster wisdom in young physicians, and she has implemented a similar program, Wisdom in Nursing, in the UVA School of Nursing. With Dorrie and Tim, she is lead author of *Self Care for Nurses: Small Doses for Wellness*. She earned a BA in economics and urban studies from Wellesley College, an MA in creative writing from Boston University, and her PhD in educational research from the UVA Curry School of Education. May lives in Richmond, Virginia, with her husband, Jim. Her most consistent and effective self-care practices are modern quilting and walking near water, especially the James River near her home and the ocean at the Outer Banks in North Carolina.

Contributing Authors

We would like to thank the following authors for their contributions to the book and their help in developing the exercises and prompts that form the essence of this facilitator guide. We appreciate their diversity of experience and viewpoints.

- Kim Acquaviva, PhD, MSW, CSE, FNAP (she/her)
- Robin C. Brown-Haithco, MDiv (she/her)
- Reynaldo "Ren" Capucao, Jr., MSN, RN, CNL (he/him)
- Theresa Carroll, PhD (she/her)
- Ebru Çayir, PhD, MD (she/her)
- Roxana Chicas, PhD, RN (she/her)
- Anna DeLong, MSW, LCSW, CEAP (she/her)
- Susan Goins-Eplee, MSN, MDiv, RN, CNL, HEC-C (she/her)
- Rosa Gonzalez-Guarda, PhD, MPH, RN, FAAN (she/her)
- Julie Haizlip, MD, MAPP (she/her)
- McKenzie Harper, MAT (she/her)
- Susan Hassmiller, PhD, RN, FAAN (she/her)
- Pamela Marie Hobby (she/her)
- Ashley R. Hurst, JD, M.Div, MA (she/her)
- Carrie McDermott, PhD, APRN, ACNS-BC (she/her)
- Elizabeth Métraux (she/her)
- Joy Miller, MSN, BS, RN, CPNP-PC, CHPPN (she/her)
- Esther Golda Lozana Otis, BSN, RN, IBCLC (she/her)
- Courtney M. Ott, DNP, MSN, BS, RN (she/her)
- Kimberly Pate, DNP, RN, ACCNS-AG, PCCN, NE-BC, FCNS (she/her)
- Arminda B. Perch, MBA, LCSW (she/her)
- Erik Pérez, OTD, OTR (he/him)
- Elizabeth A. (Lili) Powell, PhD (she/her)
- Millie Sattler, DNP, MSN, RN, CCRN (she/her)
- John Schorling, MD, MPH (he/him)
- Ryan Thomas, BSN, RN, CCRN, NRP (he/him)

Special Note to Readers

Here at Sigma, we realize that language is constantly evolving. The meaning of a word often changes over time, some words become obsolete, and some terms that were once acceptable may become controversial or even offensive, depending on the context or circumstances. We have made every effort to make language choices that are inclusive and not offensive. Should you identify words in this book that you believe negatively impact a group or groups of people, please reach out to us at Publications@SigmaNursing.org.

Table of Contents

About the Authors..iii
Contributing Authors...v
An Invitation and Welcome From the Authors..ix
About *Self-Care for New and Student Nurses*......................................x
Getting on the Same Page About Self-Care...xiv
Facilitator Resources..xvi
Introduction...xxi

section I Fundamentals 1

 1 The Fundamentals of Stress, Burnout, and Self-Care....... 2
 2 The Fundamentals of Resilience, Growth, and Wisdom ... 7
 3 Developing a Resilient Mindset Using Appreciative Practices 12

section II The Mind of a Nurse 19

 4 Self-Care, Communal Care, and Resilience Among Underrepresented Minoritized Nursing Professionals and Students... 20
 5 Self-Care for LGBTQIA+ Nursing Students 25
 6 Racial Trauma and Healing.. 29
 7 Narrative Practices... 34
 8 Self-Care and Systemic Change: What You Need to Know 39
 9 Strengths-Based Self-Care: Good Enough, Strong Enough, Wise Enough 43

section III The Body and Spirit of a Nurse 47

 10 Reclaiming, Recalling, and Remembering: Spirituality and Self-Care... 48
 11 Sleep, Exercise, and Nutrition: Self-Care the Kaizen Way 51
 12 Reflections on Self-Care and Your Clinical Practice 56

section IV The Transition to Nursing Practice 60

- 13 Supportive Professional Relationships: Nurse Residency Programs, Preceptors, and Mentors 61
- 14 Healthy Work Environment: How to Choose One for Your First Job 66
- 15 Self-Care for Humanitarian Aid Workers 71

section V The Heart of a Nurse........................75

- 16 Mattering: Creating a Rich Work Life..................... 76
- 17 Integrating a Life That Works With a Life That Counts ... 81
- 18 Providing Compassionate Care and Addressing Unmet Social Needs Can Reduce Your Burnout 85
- 19 Showing Up With Grit and Grace: How to Lead Under Pressure as a Nurse Leader 89
- 20 Coaching Yourself When Things Are Hard 93

An Invitation and Welcome From the Authors

Thank you for selecting *Self-Care for New and Student Nurses* for your course. We consider it an honor to be part of your classroom, and we hope that in choosing this text you are as committed as we are to helping nurses flourish in their newly chosen careers.

We have prepared this facilitator guide for *Self-Care for New and Student Nurses* to assist you in class preparation and to offer our thoughts and experience in teaching much of this material. The facilitator guide content parallels the activities in the *Self-Care for New and Student Nurses* workbook, providing you with a menu of classroom activities and assignments.

That said, we encourage you to rely on your own experience, creativity, and local resources to make this course as valuable as possible to your students.

Depending on the year or level of student, some topics may merit more focus than others. For example, fourth-year BSN students might want to take a deep dive into Chapter 14, "Healthy Work Environment: How to Choose One for Your First Job." If your students are expressing concern about clinician burnout or nursing shortages, you may want to spend more time with Chapter 8, "Self-Care and Systemic Change: What You Need to Know." We hope that in every chapter you will share your expertise, experiences, and wisdom with your students. Most of all, we hope you enjoy the self-care discovery process together and that your study of self-care is valuable for student and teacher alike.

About *Self-Care for New and Student Nurses*

In the *Self-Care for New and Student Nurses* introduction, we offer this invitation to our readers, your students:

> This book, we hope, will be valuable specifically to the student nurse and early career nurse. No matter where you are in your nursing trajectory, we hope that keeping your mind and body safe and strong is a high priority for you. We hope that is why you picked up this book, because you understand that the knowledge and skills you learn in school are important, but they are not all it takes to be an extraordinary nurse. You understand that your work will be challenging and that caring for yourself will help you care for others.
>
> Self-care practices are important because we need you.
>
> We need all the gifts that you bring to the nursing profession. Your future patients need you. Your future colleagues need you. We need you to become the best nurse you can possibly be so that you can support other young nurses as they, too, enter this profession. Nursing will afford you daily interactions that will change the lives of your patients, strengthen the resolve of your colleagues, and ripple beyond your immediate circle to surprising places. The gifts that you bring are beyond measure.

We have organized the book into five sections. In Section I, "Fundamentals," we provide an overview of why self-care is so important in nursing, what we mean by resilience, and concrete practices to get the reader started.

In Section II, "The Mind of a Nurse," we explore practices that address the needs of underrepresented nursing students, LGBTQIA+ students, international students, as well as narrative and mindfulness practices. This new edition also includes a chapter on racial trauma and healing with hands-on, concrete steps toward empowerment. Section II also includes an important chapter about the risks of "one-sided" resilience training, or the importance of a healthy work environment to nurses' health and well-being.

In Section III, "The Body and Spirit of a Nurse," we explore the physical and spiritual needs of the resilient nurse. We talk more about strengths-based resilience, and we bring back a popular chapter by Joy Miller about integrating well-being practices into the workday. We include a chapter on physical well-being, with a focus on sleep, exercise, and nutrition.

Section IV, "The Transition to Nursing Practice," was designed to help students navigate that anxiety-provoking period between finishing their studies and beginning their practice. What is the role of a mentor? How do you choose a healthy work environment? We even include a chapter about humanitarian aid nursing, a path that students might want to explore. We hope this section helps your students navigate this exciting, if fraught, period.

The final section, "The Heart of a Nurse," focuses on the early years of nursing. No matter where students land professionally, they will not be working alone. We hope Section V sparks ideas about ways to navigate the interpersonal, interprofessional, and organizational issues they may face.

Each chapter includes sidebars, often including vignettes, that further illustrate the chapter topic. We have also included several stand-alone essays, written by nurses from many backgrounds at various points in their careers. We find these voices of practicing nurses compelling, shining light on self-care practices in the "real world." This edition includes several new essays that we hope will spark discussion in the classroom. These were topics suggested by users of the first edition, and they include:

- The Wisdom of Nurses (advice from nurses in practice)
- Carrying Baggage: Wishing Things Were Different (mindfulness and self-compassion)
- The Expression of Authentic Cultural Self as a Form of Self-Care
- Imposter Syndrome in Nursing: "When Will I Be Enough?"
- Dopamine: How to Make It Work for You
- Making the Most of Your Journey: Flourishing in Nursing School, Clinical, and Your Nursing Career
- Research Mentorship for Social Justice and Well-Being
- What Do I Do If I Hate My First Job?
- Six Practices to Foster the "Perfect" Workday
- Making and Keeping Friends as a New Nurse

Teaching Strategies

The unique and personal nature of this course prevents us from giving you exquisitely detailed, step-by-step instructions on how to deliver the material. Our goal is to ensure that you are comfortable with the topic and that you have the materials you need to be a trusted leader for your students as they navigate this vital aspect of their future practice. Some ideas to consider:

- Given the personal nature of the material, your students will engage with *Self-Care for New and Student Nurses* and each other if they feel comfortable having honest and vulnerable conversations. You might consider establishing classroom norms at the beginning of the semester around confidentiality, respect, and active listening.

- Because the goal of this course is for students to practice self-care behaviors as regularly as possible, we encourage you to find creative ways to hold them accountable to themselves and to each other. For example, some instructors ask students, as they enter the classroom, to write one word or sentence about their self-care practice since the class last met. These could be anything: "I hate running, but walking is OK." "My dog is my best therapy." "I did better with sleep this week." You could also write a prompt on the whiteboard that differs from week to week. A gratitude board or a collection of student strengths are powerful to read. You could also create a class "positivity portfolio," asking each student to send you a photo of something that gives them joy, and then you can begin the class with a slide show. The possibilities are endless! Students will have great ideas, too.

- Identify your own self-care practices, goals, and vulnerabilities. It is important for you to model self-care behaviors and to be able to speak honestly about the challenges you struggle with. If self-care is not your strong suit, we encourage you to be honest about that with your students but commit to learning and practicing with them.

- Take the opportunity to visualize your goals for this class. What would be your ideal outcome at the end of the semester? Will it be more empowered students who feel confident about their ability to maintain their well-being during their first year of clinical practice? Is it students who feel connected to one another in a deeper, more meaningful way? Dream big. Imagine your goals in as much detail as possible. (Are students laughing together? Do they show kindness toward one another? In what specific ways? Are they advocating for their fellow students' well-being to school administrators?) As we describe in Chapter 3, positive visualization is a powerful tool.

- There are also numerous shared themes across chapters. We strived to present a wide array of self-care concepts, but you will probably notice that there are common threads that weave throughout the chapters, and we call this "synergy." You may also notice some redundancy. If you see a topic or idea multiple times, please assume that it is something we think is very important. As Jon Kabat-Zinn (2010) said, "There are a million doors into the same room." We hope your students will try opening as many doors, and try as many practices, as time will allow.

- Finally, take care of yourself as you take this journey with your students. Have fun. Laugh. Try new things. Be creative. Ask your colleagues for help. Let conversations and class discussions go where they go.

Thoughts on Assignments

Homework: The *Self-Care for New and Student Nurses* workbook contains activities for each chapter. These are structured in a *What-Why-Do-Reflect & Journal* format. Although it is important for students to learn the didactic material, it is even more important for them to practice the self-care techniques and have the opportunity to process them. They should have the opportunity to process the material in the *Reflect & Journal* activities and in classroom discussion with you and their peers. We think that journal assignments should remain personal to each student, but you may want to periodically ask for reflection papers that they know will be turned in to you or shared with other students.

Classroom activities: Many classroom discussions can begin with prompts from the workbook, and we have added several activities and classroom discussion questions in this facilitator guide. Discussions can be done in pairs, small groups, or as an entire classroom.

Course assignment #1: Research Paper: We recommend asking students to do a deep dive into at least one self-care practice or topic over the course of the semester. This would potentially include writing a research paper on the topic; trying to do the practice, when feasible; and presenting their research and personal experience to the class. Their findings could become part of their own or their peers' self-care toolkit.

Potential research topics (and this is the tip of the iceberg):

Pet therapy	Reiki	Moral distress
Coping with bullying in nursing	Sleep hygiene	Mindfulness
Mental health stigma in health-care professions	How to train for a marathon	Substance use disorders among practicing nurses
Yoga	Health benefits of walking	How to breathe
Art therapy	Health benefits of social connections	Gratitude practices
Humor therapy	Nurses' health study	Burnout
Music therapy	Harvard study of adult development	Compassion
Dialectical behavior therapy	Impact of COVID-19 pandemic on nurses' well-being	Narrative practices

Course assignment #2: Self-Care Toolkit: We hope that every student will engage in many self-care practices during the course and evaluate which are effective for them, which they might modify for their own lifestyle and preferences, and which might be more useful in the future. In each workbook chapter, we encourage students to use the *Reflect & Journal* assignments to consider their personal toolkit. We encourage you to engage with students about their progress in creating their toolkit. This can be in the form of regular written assignments or a product at the end of the course.

Getting on the Same Page About Self-Care

There are some harmful myths when it comes to self-care. What comes to mind when you hear the words "self-care"? Does the idea of caring for yourself sound selfish? Do you think of a good night's sleep, a meal that includes a vegetable, or a workout at the gym? Is self-care something you'll do later, when you're in the throes of a stressful nursing job? Is self-care all up to you, something you alone can address?

We want to address these myths before going any further:

- Self-care is not selfish. Nurses should be entitled, in fact expected, to care for themselves with the same creativity and compassion that they use to care for others.

- Nurses don't flourish simply by fostering the well-being of others. The nursing profession is inherently meaningful in that we care for patients and families during their most vulnerable moments. But meaningful work has its limits. A major thread throughout this book is that we don't want to be "the naked person offering someone their coat."

- Self-care is about the mind as much as it is about the body. Yes, sleep, exercise, and good nutrition are important. But self-care involves how we harness the gift of brain neuroplasticity, mindfulness, and our ability to pay attention to ourselves and others.

- Self-care is a lifelong *practice*, and it is best to begin the practice early, before facing the stressors of a hospital or other clinical setting. In general, nursing students face significantly more stress than their peers, increasing the importance and value of self-care practices during nursing school.

- Individual self-care practices do not let organizations off the hook. The importance of a healthy work environment cannot be overstated, and in this book, we offer help in selecting a healthy workplace and encourage readers to advocate for themselves and others.

What Is Self-Care?

Nursing researchers Pam Ashcraft and Susan Gatto (2018, p. 140) offer that self-care "can be described as deliberate decisions made and actions taken by individuals to address their own health and well-being." We appreciate their emphasis on "deliberate decisions" and the recognition that we are all empowered to manage our behaviors and resulting health and well-being. This is an excellent starting point.

This book contains many voices, and we hope diversity strengthens the power of this work. We noticed in final edits that there were many more similarities across the chapters than we realized. We find it reassuring to know that so many experts on self-care and resilience point to similar strategies. The authors often come to the same place but from different perspectives, sometimes using different language and frameworks. Again, we hope these variations allow each student to find the voice that best speaks to them.

With this diversity, we have been able to include many tools, ideas, and paths to well-being in the text, but if we had to give you two goals for your teaching, they would be these:

- We have the power to choose—our focus, our response to stimuli around us, and the deliberate decisions we make for our own health and well-being.
- We cannot care compassionately for ourselves and others unless we master the art of paying attention. There are many explanations of the value of paying attention throughout the book, and we highlighted many of them in this facilitator guide.

references

Ashcraft, P. F., & Gatto, S. L. (2018). Curricular interventions to promote self-care in prelicensure nursing students. *Nurse Educator, 43*(3), 140–144. https://doi.org/10.1097/NNE.0000000000000450

Kabat-Zinn, J. (2010, March). *Mindfulness in medicine and psychology: Its transformative and healing potential in living and in dying*. Talk presented at the University of Virginia.

Facilitator Resources

You will notice that most chapters come with extensive bibliographies, and we encourage you to take a deeper dive into topics that you or your students gravitate toward. We also asked our contributors to tell us which additional books or articles were important to their work; we have included them in the list that follows.

Introduction

Ashcraft, P. F., & Gatto, S. L. (2018). Curricular interventions to promote self-care in prelicensure nursing students, *Nurse Educator, 43*(3), 140–144. https://doi.org/10.1097/NNE.0000000000000450

Kabat-Zinn, J. (2010, March). *Mindfulness in medicine and psychology: Its transformative and healing potential in living and in dying.* Talk presented at the University of Virginia, Virginia, U.S.

Lazenby, M. (2017). *Caring matters most: The ethical significance of nursing.* Oxford University Press.

Mackesy, C. (2019). *The boy, the mole, the fox and the horse.* HarperCollins.

Chapter 1: The Fundamentals of Stress, Burnout, and Self-Care

Halifax, J. (2018). *Standing at the edge: Facing freedom where fear and courage meet.* Flatiron Books.

Lorde, A. (2017). *A burst of light and other essays.* Dover.

Nagoski, E., & Nagoski, A. (2019). *Burnout: The secret to unlocking the stress cycle.* Ballantine Books.

Taylor, J. B. (2008). *My stroke of insight: A brain scientist's personal journey.* Penguin Books.

Chapter 2: The Fundamentals of Resilience, Growth, and Wisdom

Achor, S. (2010). *The happiness advantage: The seven principles of positive psychology that fuel success and performance at work.* Crown Business.

Brown, B. (2012). *Daring greatly: How the courage to be vulnerable transforms the way we live, love, parent, and lead.* Gotham House.

Brown, B. (2017). *Braving the wilderness: The quest for true belonging and the courage to stand alone.* Random House.

Diener, E., & Biswas-Diener, R. (2008). *Happiness: Unlocking the mysteries of psychological wealth.* Blackwell Publishing.

Doyle, G. (2020). *Untamed.* The Dial Press.

Hanson, R. (2018). *Resilient: How to grow an unshakable core of calm, strength, and happiness.* Harmony Books.

Irvine, W. B. (2009). *A guide to the good life: The ancient art of Stoic joy.* Oxford University Press, Inc.

Irvine, W. B. (2019). *The Stoic challenge: A philosopher's guide to becoming tougher, calmer, and more resilient.* W. W. Norton & Co., Inc.

Schwartz, B., & Sharpe, K. (2010). *Practical wisdom: The right way to do the right thing.* Riverhead Books.

Thaler, R. H., & Sunstein, C.R. (2009). *Nudge: Improving decisions about health, wealth, and happiness.* Penguin Books.

Chapter 3: Developing a Resilient Mindset Using Appreciative Practices

Frankl, V. (2006). *Man's search for meaning.* Beacon Press.

Hanson, R. (2013). *Hardwiring happiness: The new brain science of contentment, calm, and confidence.* Harmony Books.

Kelm, J. B. (2005). *Appreciative living: The principles of appreciative inquiry in personal life.* Venet Publishers.

Kross, E. (2021). *Chatter: The voice in our head, why it matters, and how to harness it.* Crown.

Lee, I. F. (2018). *Joyful: The surprising power of ordinary things to create extraordinary happiness.* Little, Brown Spark.

Chapter 4: Self-Care, Communal Care, and Resilience Among Underrepresented Minoritized Nursing Professionals and Students

Flanagan, D. (2020). *Dream big and awaken to your possibilities*. Flanagan Publishing.

Gardner, J. (2005). Barriers influencing the success of racial and ethnic minority students in nursing programs. *Journal of Transcultural Nursing, 16*(2), 155–162. https://doi.org/10.1177/1043659604273546

Zambrana, R. (2018). *Toxic ivory towers: The consequences of work stress on underrepresented minority faculty*. Rutgers University Press.

Chapter 5: Self-Care for LGBTQIA+ Nursing Students

Avery-Desmarais, S., Sethares, K. A., Stover, C., Batchelder, A., & McCurry, M. K. (2020). Substance use and minority stress in a population of lesbian, gay and bisexual nurses. *Substance Use & Misuse, 55*(12), 1958–1967. https://doi.org/10.1080/10826084.2020.1784946

Bell, B. (2021). Towards abandoning the master's tools: The politics of a universal nursing identity. *Nursing Inquiry, 28*(2), e12395. https://doi.org/10.1111/nin.12395

Blackwell, C. W., Diaz-Cruz, A., & Yan, X. (2020). Equality and quality: The relationship between Magnet® status and healthcare organizational commitment to lesbian, gay, bisexual, and transgender equality. *Journal of Social Service Research, 46*(2), 1–8. https://doi.org/10.1080/01488376.2019.1645796

Braun, H. M., Ramirez, D., Zahner, G. J., Gillis-Buck, E. M., Sheriff, H., & Ferrone, M. (2017). The LGBTQI health forum: An innovative interprofessional initiative to support curriculum reform. *Medical Education Online, 22*(1), 1306419. https://doi.org/10.1080/10872981.2017.1306419

Eliason, M. J., DeJoseph, J., Dibble, S., Deevey, S., & Chinn, P. (2011). Lesbian, gay, bisexual, transgender, and queer/questioning nurses' experiences in the workplace. *Journal of Professional Nursing, 27*, 237–244. https://doi.org/10.1016/j.profnurs.2011.03.003

Eliason, M., Streed, C., & Henne, M. (2018). Coping with stress as an LGBTQ+ health care professional. *Journal of Homosexuality, 65*(5), 561–578. https://doi.org/10.1080/00918369.2017.1328224

Kroning, M. (2018). Lesbian, gay, bisexual, and transgender education in nursing. *Nurse Educator, 43*(1), 41. https://doi.org/10.1097/NNE.0000000000000429

Meyer, I. H. (2015). Resilience in the study of minority stress and health of sexual and gender minorities. *Psychology of Sexual Orientation and Gender Diversity, 2*(3), 209–213. https://doi.org/10.1037/sgd0000132

Morrow, M. R., & Avery-Desmarais, S. (2024). Follow your passion and discover the beauty of being a nurse scientist. *Nursing Science Quarterly, 37*(1), 29–32. https://doi.org/10.1177/08943184231207369

Nadal, K. L., Wong, Y., Issa, M. A., Meterko, V., Leon, J., & Wideman, M. (2011). Sexual orientation microaggressions: Processes and coping mechanisms for lesbian, gay, and bisexual individuals. *Journal of LGBT Issues in Counseling, 5*(1), 21–46. https://doi.org/10.1080/15538605.2011.554606

Przedworski, J. M., Dovidio, J. F., Hardeman, R. R., Phelan, S. M., Burke, S. E., Ruben, M. A., Perry, S. P., Burgess, D. J., Nelson, D. B., Yeazel, M. W., Knudsen, J. M., & van Ryn, M. (2015). A comparison of the mental health and well-being of sexual minority and heterosexual first-year medical students: A report from the medical student CHANGE Study. *Academic Medicine, 90*(5), 652–658. https://doi.org/10.1097/acm.0000000000000658

Sánchez, N. F., Rankin, S., Callahan, E., Ng, H., Holaday, L., McIntosh, K., Poll-Hunter, N., & Sánchez, J. P. (2015). LGBT trainee and health professional perspectives on academic careers—Facilitators and challenges. *LGBT Health, 2*(4), 346–356. https://doi.org/10.1089/lgbt.2015.0024

Sandfort, T. G. M., Bakker, F., Schellevis, F., & Vanwesenbeeck, I. (2009). Coping styles as mediator of sexual orientation-related health. *Archives of Sexual Behavior, 38*(2), 253–263. https://doi.org/10.1007/s10508-007-9233-9

Sitkin, N. A., & Pachankis, J. E. (2016). Specialty choice among sexual and gender minorities in medicine: The role of specialty prestige, perceived inclusion, and medical school climate. *LGBT Health, 3*(6), 451–460. https://doi.org/10.1089/lgbt.2016.0058

Soled, K. R., Clark, K. D., Altman, M. R., Bosse, J. D., Thompson, R. A., Squires, A., & Sherman, A. D. (2022). Changing language, changes lives: Learning the lexicon of LGBTQ+ health equity. *Research in Nursing & Health, 45*(6), 621–632. https://doi.org/10.1002/nur.22274

Toomey, R. B., Ryan, C., Diaz, R. M., & Russell, S. T. (2018). Coping with sexual orientation—Related minority stress. *Journal of Homosexuality, 65*(4), 484–500. https://doi.org/10.1080/00918369.2017.1321888

Zollweg, S. S. F., Tobin, V., Goldstein, Z. G., Keepnews, D. M., & Chinn, P. L. (2020). Improving LGBTQ+ health: Nursing policy can make a difference. *Policy & Politics in Nursing and Health Care-E-Book*, 211.

Chapter 6: Racial Trauma and Healing

Hardy, K. V. (2023). *Racial trauma: Clinical strategies & techniques for healing invisible wounds*. W. W. Norton & Company.

Rowe, S. W. (2020). *Healing racial trauma: The road to resilience*. IVP.

Williams, M. T. (2020) *Managing microaggresions*. Oxford University Press.

Chapter 11: Sleep, Exercise, and Nutrition: Self-Care the Kaizen Way

Nester, J. (2020). *Breath: The new science of a lost art*. Riverhead Books.

Walker, M. (2017). *Why we sleep: Unlocking the power of sleep and dreams*. Scribner.

Chapter 14: Healthy Work Environment: How to Choose One for Your First Job

Alspach, G. (2016). The toxic wake of rudeness: Why it matters. *Critical Care Nursing, 36(5)*, 10–13. https://doi.org/10.4037/ccn2016762

Porath, C. (2016). *Mastering civility: A manifesto for the workplace*. Grand Central Publishing.

Salzberg, S. (1995). *Lovingkindness: The revolutionary arc of happiness*. Shambala Publications.

Salzberg, S. (2014). *Real happiness at work: Meditations for accomplishment, achievement, and peace*. Workman Publishing.

White, K. R., & Fontaine, D. K. (2017). *Boost your nursing leadership career: 50 lessons that drive success*. Health Administration Press.

Worline, M. C., & Dutton, J. E. (2017). *Awakening compassion at work: The quiet power that elevates people and organizations*. Berrett-Koehler Publishers.

Chapter 16: Mattering: Creating a Rich Work Life

Flett, G. L. (2018). *The psychology of mattering: Understanding the human need to be significant*. Elsevier Inc.

Wambach, A. (2019). *Wolfpack: How to come together, unleash our power, and change the game*. Celadon Books.

Chapter 17: Integrating a Life That Works With a Life That Counts

Achor, S. (2010). *The happiness advantage: The seven principles of positive psychology that fuel success and performance at work*. Crown Business.

Bauer-Wu, S. (2011). *Leaves falling gently: Living fully with serious and life-limiting illness through mindfulness, compassion and connectedness*. New Harbinger Publications.

Cuddy, A. (2015). *Presence: Bringing your boldest self to your biggest challenges*. Back Bay Books.

Heath, C., & Heath, D. (2017). *The power of moments: Why certain experiences have extraordinary impact*. Simon & Schuster.

Chapter 18: Providing Compassionate Care and Addressing Unmet Social Needs Can Reduce Your Burnout

Bowler, K. (2018). *Everything happens for a reason: And other lies I've loved*. Random House.

Cahalan, S. (2013). *Brain on fire: My month of madness*. Simon and Schuster.

Dempsey, C. (2018). *The antidote to suffering: How compassionate connected care can improve safety, quality, and experience*. Press Ganey Associates.

Hassmiller, S. (2020). *Resetting: An unplanned journey of loss, love, and living again*. Morgan James Publishing.

The National Academy of Medicine. (2021). *A second report on the future of nursing*. National Academies Press.

Price, R. (2000). *A whole new life*. Simon and Schuster.

Yip-Williams, J. (2020). *The unwinding of the miracle: A memoir of life, death, and everything that comes after*. Random House Trade Paperbacks.

Chapter 19: Showing Up With Grit and Grace: How to Lead Under Pressure as a Nurse Clinician and Leader

Bergland, C. (2013, Feb. 2). The neurobiology of grace under pressure. *Psychology Today*. https://www.psychologytoday.com/us/blog/the-athletes-way/201302/the-neurobiology-grace-under-pressure

Cuddy, A., Kohut, M., & Neffinger, J. (2013). Connect, then lead. *Harvard Business Review*. https://hbr.org/2013/07/connect-then-lead

Duckworth, A. (2016). *Grit: The power of passion and perseverance*. Scribner.

Halpern, B. L., & Lubar, K. (2004). *Leadership presence: Dramatic techniques to reach out, motivate and inspire*. Gotham.

Hanson, R. (2018). *Resilient: Find your inner strength*. Rider.

Hougaard, R., & Carter, J. (2018). *The mind of the leader: How to lead yourself, your people, and your organization for extraordinary results*. Harvard Business Review Press.

Powell, L., & Hunter, J. (2020, June 26). How to recapture leadership's lost moment. *Leader to Leader*. https://doi.org/10.1002/ltl.20519

Trzeciak, S., & Mazzarelli, A. (2019). *Compassionomics: The revolutionary scientific evidence that caring makes a difference*. Studer Group.

Worline, M., & Dutton, J. (2017). *Awakening compassion at work: The quiet power that elevates people and organizations*. Berrett-Koehler.

Chapter 20: Coaching Yourself When Things Are Hard

Gay, R. (2022). *The book of delights*. Algonquin Books of Chapel Hill.

Introduction

In the textbook's introduction, we talk about the influence that nurses have on others, their superpower of compassion that they may never even be aware of. We write:

> Imagine for a moment a patient who is a young mother. Perhaps she is facing her health challenges while trying to be strong for her children and partner. The kindness, wisdom, and support that you bring to your interactions with her will have a downstream impact on her children and family. Even her children's children. Think about yourself or your nursing school peers who, when asked why they wanted to become a nurse, tell a story about growing up and seeing a nurse who cared for them or a loved one during a health crisis. So many nurses are nurses because they experienced the compassion of someone like you when they were in need. These nurses' compassion may have started you on your own journey to nursing, even though they may never know the impact they had on you. That is one of the superpowers of nursing: the impact you have on others. *You will matter* in ways big and small, in ways that the universe may never even be able to reveal to you.

This would be an appropriate time to ask students to share their path to nursing and to remember those who influenced their decision to become a nurse. Depending on their level of experience, you could invite them to reflect on times when they felt as if they mattered to a patient, a patient's family, or a colleague. The goal of this exercise is both to underscore the impact of our behavior on others (good and bad, but in this case, good) and to reflect on the superpower of compassion embodied in nursing.

Ask students how they define self-care:

- What does it mean to you?
- What comes to mind when you hear the term?
- Why did you choose to enroll in this course (if it is an elective)? What do you hope to gain from this course?

The goal of this discussion is to sort through myths about self-care as we described in the "Getting on the Same Page About Self-Care" section earlier. (This material also appears in the textbook's introduction and the workbook introduction.) We hope that students begin to understand that:

- Self-care is not selfish.
- Nurses don't flourish simply by fostering the well-being of others.
- Self-care is about the mind as much as it is about the body.
- Self-care is a lifelong practice, and it is best to begin the practice before facing the stressors of a hospital or other clinical setting.
- Individual self-care practices do not let organizations off the hook.

Stanford Medicine, WellMD, and WellPhD released a powerful five-minute video in 2024 that honors the shared humanity of health workers, *I Am Human*. You might consider sharing this video with your students to prompt discussion: https://www.youtube.com/watch?v=QCZCiZ0K57M

section I
Fundamentals

1
The Fundamentals of Stress, Burnout, and Self-Care

–Natalie May

what

Read Chapter 1.

- What do we mean by the phrase "a naked person offering someone their shirt"?

  It's from the opening quote by Maya Angelou: "I do not trust people who don't love themselves and yet tell me, 'I love you.' There is an African saying which is: Be careful when a naked person offers you a shirt." Nurses are often the ones caring for others but not caring as well for themselves. *Self-Care for New and Student Nurses,* 2nd Edition, is an invitation to not be that naked person.

- Describe the differences between stress, stressors, and burnout.

  Stress is anything that causes a sudden physical or psychological reaction.

  Stressors are the stressful situations that result in stress. There are good and bad stressors, from exams and sports competitions to physical danger and trauma.

  Burnout is an employee's response to excessive work-related stress—stress that goes unaddressed for a long period of time. It is not a result of a one-time stressor. It stems from one or more "mismatches" between an employee and their work. Burnout can have physical and behavioral symptoms. Maslach conceptualized burnout as having three dimensions: emotional exhaustion, depersonalization, and reduced sense of personal accomplishment (Maslach, 1998; Maslach & Jackson, 1981).

- List five stressors that nurses face in the workplace that are unique to healthcare and nursing.

High workload	Poor supervisor/leader support
Low staffing levels	Poor leadership
Long shifts	Negative team relationship
Low control	Job insecurity
Low schedule flexibility	Lifting/repositioning heavy objects
Time pressure	Physical assault by patient or patient's family
High job and psychological demands	
Low task variety	Concerns for physical safety
Role conflict	Musculoskeletal pain at work
Low autonomy	Coming in early/staying late/working through breaks
Negative nurse-physician relationship	Bullying

> Working more than 10 hours/day
>
> Busy, complex work environment
>
> Routinely confronting human suffering, patient morbidity, and mortality
>
> Complex ethical decision-making
>
> Difficult conversations with patients and families
>
> Work-family conflict
>
> Societal stressors, such as aging of baby boomers, physician shortages, nursing shortages, uncertainties of healthcare reform, COVID-19 pandemic

- Why are new and early-career nurses more vulnerable to burnout and stress-related ill health than more experienced nurses?

  - Stress of being in a new role
  - Having to master new skills in a high-stakes environment
  - Socialization into a new profession and workplace
  - Heavy workloads
  - Unsupportive practice environments
  - Daily work not matching expectations

- What barriers to self-care might you face as a practicing nurse?

  - Not enough time/being overworked
  - Lack of adequate resources and facilities
  - Fatigue/lack of sleep
  - Outside commitments, such as family, community, attending school
  - Unhealthy food culture

why

- List three reasons a personal self-care practice is important for nurses.

  > This prompt is a good class discussion question and will provide students an opportunity to discuss compassionate care goals as well as their own well-being and personal goals.

- List three reasons a personal self-care practice is important *to you*.

> This prompt is intended to allow students an opportunity to identify their own professional and personal goals. You may also want to invite them to share the stressors they face. These could include struggles to get enough exercise or sleep, manage anxiety, or set and maintain boundaries.

do

Activity 1-1: My Current Self-Care Practice Inventory

- We are quite certain that you already engage in self-care practices, whether you label them as such or not. Think back over the past few years. What do you do to care for yourself when you feel stressed, anxious, or overwhelmed? Do you go for a run? Call a friend? Knit? Knock back a few beers? Do some online shopping? Write down all the activities that you turn to when you need to calm yourself.

- Once you have made this list, put a plus sign next to the activities that you think are helpful and that you would like to include in your self-care toolkit. Put a minus sign next to those that you might want to eliminate or modify, such as self-medicating with food or drink.

Activity 1-2: Self-Care Google Exploration

- This activity is included in the textbook. Google the terms "self-care" and "self-care practices." Expand your search if you're feeling especially ambitious or curious.

- Make a list of some of what pops up. You will find memes, posters, infographics, quotes, research articles, and more. Make a list, or a Pinterest board, of things that intrigue you or resonate with your personality and current self-care practices.

- Which concepts make you think, "I could get into this," or, "This makes sense to me"? What ideas intrigue you or make you want to learn more? These concepts might be your own personal entrées into the study and practice of self-care.

- As you are browsing the internet for self-care practices and ideas, try to categorize each practice into one of the following self-care and wellness categories: physical, mental, emotional, spiritual, intellectual, social, financial, and environmental. Some may fit into more than one category.

> We address this later in *Self-Care for New and Student Nurses*, but it may come up in this discussion: #selfcare, or toxic presentations of self-care practices, might make students feel inadequate or excluded due to their social or economic backgrounds or for other reasons. Welcome this discussion and how it will factor into their personal exploration of self-care.

Activity 1-3: Try the Big Four

We end Chapter 1 with four of the fundamental self-care practices: staying hydrated; checking in with yourself and unclenching when you find tension in your body; taking deep, restorative breaths; and staying present. Begin to integrate these practices into your daily routine. Use whatever reminder system works best for you, whether it's alarms on your phone, post-it notes, or something else.

reflect & journal

- As you explore self-care practices in your Google search, try to imagine yourself engaging in some of these practices. Are you an athlete or an artist? Do you recoup your energy by being in nature? Is your highest priority staying connected with family and friends?

- What self-care practices would you like to learn more about and consider including in your self-care toolkit?

- Which of the Big Four practices (hydration, unclenching, breathing, being present) come most naturally to you? Which ones will take a little more work? Why?

- As you begin this journey, we want to caution you about comparing yourself to others. Comparing ourselves to others can often feel like a competition and can induce more stress and self-doubt. As you journal about your experiences with self-care, consider a different type of comparison. Compare yourself not to others, but to you. Observe the progress you have made. Celebrate your curiosity and willingness to try new things. Stick to it. Ask for help when you need it. Support and acknowledge the progress of others.

references

Maslach, C. (1998). A multidimensional theory of burnout. In C. L. Cooper (Ed.), *Theories of organizational stress* (pp. 68–85). Oxford University Press Inc.

Maslach, C., & Jackson, S. E. (1981). The measurement of experienced burnout. *Journal of Organizational Behavior, 2*, 99–113. https://doi.org/10.1002/job.4030020205

2
The Fundamentals of Resilience, Growth, and Wisdom

–Natalie May

what

Read Chapter 2.

- What do we mean by the term "resilience"?

  - The ability to bounce back from adversity; the capacity to recover from adversity or trauma

  - A trait that helps nurses and others avoid the effects of unmitigated workplace stress, or burnout

  Mental resources like determination, self-worth, and kindness are what make us *resilient*: able to cope with adversity and push through challenges in pursuit of opportunities. Although resilience helps us recover from loss and trauma, it offers much more than that. True resilience fosters well-being, an underlying sense of happiness, love, and peace. Remarkably, as you internalize experiences of well-being, it builds inner strengths that in turn make you more resilient. Well-being and resilience promote each other in an upward spiral (Hanson, 2018, p. 2).

  Resilience is in everyone; we have the capacity to nurture it and be mindful of its power.

- List three ways that your workplace can foster individual resilience.

  Your personal resilience skill development plus organizational support are the two primary ingredients that will determine how you respond to the stressors in your work and life. Your workplace can foster resilience with the following supports (adapted from Cusack et al., 2016):

  Policies and structures that enable a nurse to act ethically and respectfully and benefit patient care: Explicit lines of communication; receptive, responsive, understanding, supportive leadership; timely access to support for ethical guidance; and respectful working relationships

  Processes that enable nurses to deliver competent, patient-centered care: Explicit but flexible role expectations; appropriate patient allocation; availability of essential and properly working equipment; and support of interprofessional collaboration

  Practices that enable nurses to feel connected, safe, and well: Culture of kindness and positive staff behaviors; planned and monitored meal breaks; Employee Assistance Programs; and physical space for mindfulness, breathing, and meditation practices

  Opportunities for nurses to engage in reflection, career development, and lifelong learning: Mentoring programs; review processes that promote staged knowledge and skill development; and study leave

Opportunities to enhance clinical nursing practice: Practice development opportunities around clinical knowledge, skills, and problem-solving; clinical supervision systems that build competence and confidence; opportunities to debrief and learn from mistakes rather than blaming

Opportunities for nurses to learn resilience skills: Adaptive coping learning opportunities; mindfulness and meditation training

- What are the four components of grit, another kind of resilience?

    1. **Interest:** "I love what I do" feeling
    2. **Practice:** Our ability to avoid complacency, to build upward from our current skill level
    3. **Purpose:** The sense that your work matters to others (see more in Chapter 20)
    4. **Hope:** The belief that you have the power to make things better

This section begins with the question, "What do you think matters more in life: talent or hard work?" This might generate an interesting class discussion. Ask for examples of when students have succeeded through grit or have seen others do so. It is a valuable reminder to students that they have persevered in the past and have the capacity to do so now and in the future.

why

- Why is neuroplasticity important in our ability to become resilient?

    Many connections between self-care and resilience abide in the science of *neuroplasticity*, your nervous system's ability to change and form new neural pathways. This process is literally the rewiring of your brain, based on your experiences. If you have studied the effects of trauma, you know that traumatic events can change victims' brains in a negative way. Similarly, positive neuroplasticity explains why fostering your own well-being today can have a powerful impact on your well-being months or even years from now when you face adversity. By watching a funny movie or snuggling with your canine or feline companion, you are on your way to building new positive pathways in your brain. Hanson (2018) calls this the ability to "turn passing experiences into lasting inner resources built into your brain" (p. 2).

    According to Hanson (2018), the most important method of fostering resilience is to *internalize experiences of well-being.*

- In this chapter, we present two nursing students, Nevin and Pat. Explain in your own words how these two students have learned to approach challenges. Which student do you most closely resemble? Why?

do

Activity 2-1: Foster Positive Emotions

One foundation of well-being is fostering positive emotions. Just as a steady diet of negativity will breed negativity, engaging in activities that make us feel good will help us feel good. Happiness and well-being researcher Barbara Frederickson (Cohn et al., 2009) identified 10 universal positive emotions that we ask you to explore here. For this activity, write down at least one activity or experience that gives rise to each emotion in you. For example, you might feel awe when you see a hawk fly overhead. Perhaps you feel inspiration when you observe an experienced nurse perform a difficult procedure. After identifying what creates positive emotions, the next step is to be intentional about experiencing them. If calling your best friend generates feelings of love, call your best friend more often. If a particular song makes you feel joyful, listen to that song!

Emotion	Activity
Joy	
Gratitude	
Serenity	
Interest	
Hope	
Pride	
Amusement	
Inspiration	
Awe	
Love	

Activity 2-2: Savor the Moment

Rick Hanson (2018) argues that we must "sit with" positive emotions to rewire our brains for resilience. In Chapter 2, we provided a hypothetical list of daily opportunities to savor positive emotions. For at least one day, be very intentional about savoring positive moments, from the moment you wake up until you fall asleep at night. Write down as many of these moments as possible. After this one-day exercise, remind yourself to continue savoring positive emotions.

reflect & journal

- How will you be able to maintain this practice of fostering positive emotions and savoring them once you are in clinical practice? What techniques and strategies can you use to help build these activities into your daily and weekly routine?

- We all know someone, either personally or from the news or history books, who has overcome extreme adversity and grown wiser as a result of their experience. In the textbook, we include Congressman John Lewis, Malala Yousafzai, and the Marjorie Stoneman Douglas High School students as examples of individuals who were able to transform their pain into wisdom. Who do you know that you would consider wise? Why do you consider them to be wise? What qualities do they exhibit? Did they overcome adversity as part of their journey to wisdom?

- How does it feel to be intentional about fostering and savoring positive emotions? Is this a new experience for you? Is it something that you can continue to do? Why or why not?

- You are capable. You are strong. You are wise. You will become more able, strong, and wise as you learn and grow. Say it aloud to yourself: "I am capable. I am strong. I am wise." Believe it.

references

Cohn, M. A., Fredrickson, B. L., Brown, S. L., Mikels, J. A., & Conway, A. M. (2009). Happiness unpacked: Positive emotions increase life satisfaction by building resilience. *Emotion, 9*(3), 361–368. https://doi.org/10.1037/a0015952

Cusack, L., Smith, M., Hegney, D., Rees, C. S., Breen, L. J., Witt, R. R., Rogers, C., Williams, A., Cross, W., & Cheung, K. (2016). Exploring environmental factors in nursing workplaces that promote psychological resilience: Constructing a unified theoretical model. *Frontiers in Psychology, 7*, 600. https://doi.org/10.3389/fpsyg.2016.00600

Hanson, R. (2018). *Resilient: How to grow an unshakable core of calm, strength, and happiness.* Harmony Books.

3
Developing a Resilient Mindset Using Appreciative Practices

–Natalie May & Julie Haizlip

what

Read Chapter 3.

- What is the negativity bias? Give some examples of this bias in your own life.

  > As humans, and certainly as healthcare professionals, we are prone to a negativity bias (Haizlip et al., 2012). The *negativity bias* is an evolutionary construct that results in our human tendency to be more strongly influenced by the negative aspects of our environment than the positive (Baumeister et al., 2001). This makes sense from a survival perspective: It's more imperative to notice the hungry predator than the lovely sunset. The negativity bias has remained with us and affected our behaviors in numerous realms, including learning, attention, and how we make sense of the world around us (Baumeister et al., 2001; Vaish et al., 2008). The negativity bias leads us to focus on what is broken or what needs to be fixed.
  >
  > Some examples of this bias could include the following:
  > - When I receive good news, I immediately think about what could go wrong.
  > - I tend to notice what people do wrong, rather than what they do right.
  > - I tend to assume the worst in people.
  > - I don't give myself a break; I only notice what I do wrong.
  > - My parents never celebrated my good grades; they only criticized the less-than-good grades.

- What are some of the well-being benefits of positive activities?
  - Allows us to focus on what we want in ourselves and those around us, while growing the thoughts, feelings, and behaviors that support well-being and happiness
  - Supports overall health and success
  - Benefits our immune systems and cardiovascular health
  - Fosters creativity, improves cognition, reduces depression, and increases our ability to cope with stress
  - Allows us to create more of what we want more of by shifting our focus to that
  - Increases our ability to offer emotional support to others
  - In healthcare, improves decision-making and patient safety

- Explain two of the theoretical principles (constructionist, poetic, positive, simultaneity, anticipatory) of Appreciative Inquiry in your own words.

> **Constructionist principle:** Our realities are created by our thoughts, language, and interactions with others (language with care).
>
> **Poetic principle:** There is beauty in everything; it just depends on how you look at it (reframing).
>
> **Positive principle:** We are more creative, better able to solve problems, and more open to learning and to new ideas when we are experiencing positive emotions; positivity also results in social bonding (gratitude practice).
>
> **Simultaneity principle:** Our questions are fateful; change and our questions are inextricably linked (assumption of positive intent).
>
> **Anticipatory principle:** We move toward the image of the future that we hold in our heads; the more positive that vision, the more positive our future (visualization).

why

In this chapter, the authors discuss the importance of "choosing our focus." Explain what this entails and why it matters. (You may want to refer back to the Nevin and Pat examples in Chapter 2.)

> This question is intended as a reminder not only of the importance of choosing our focus but also of our own agency in improving our well-being. Many of the exercises in this chapter and Chapter 4 teach small behavior changes that improve well-being on their own but also build the "muscle" of choosing our focus and paying attention in the moment. These real-world mindfulness activities are the foundation of self-care practices.

do

Activity 3-1: Choose Language With Care

As the authors explain, language creates our reality. Observe the choices that people make with language. How does naming something a certain way change the words' impact? Pay attention to your own language choices. Did you learn to use certain words in your childhood that seem problematic today?

> This can be an opportunity to look at language in healthcare. Why do we use one term instead of another? What connotation do these words convey? (Drug addiction vs.

> substance use disorder; diabetic vs. person with diabetes; and cultural competency vs. cultural humility are a few examples.) As we wrote this book, the term "student nurse" versus "nursing student" came up a lot. What is the difference in these two terms? Here is a link to an interesting essay about this: https://nursemanifest.com/2016/04/06/nursing-students-or-student-nurses-whats-in-a-name/
>
> Encourage students to look at how language is used in the world around them—their school of nursing, their university, their communities. Language in the news always generates good discussion (e.g., illegal alien vs. immigrant vs. refugee; pro-choice vs. pro-life; etc.).

Activity 3-2: Reframing

What we choose to focus on becomes our fate (Whitney & Trosten-Bloom, 2003). *Reframing* is the capacity to intentionally explore new ways of seeing to experience the best of what is. Think of something that is annoying, sad, disappointing, or challenging. Now reframe this situation to find the best of what is. For example, you may have a long walk to your campus or hospital. You could reframe this by realizing that the walk is an opportunity for exercise, time to listen to music, or a chance to prepare for or decompress from your day.

> Literally anything can be reframed, and how we think about something determines how we feel about it. After a week of rainy days, a colleague was walking to work, grumbling to herself about the weather. She noticed an extraordinary growth of mushrooms near the sidewalk. She got out her camera, got down on the ground, and snapped photos. People stopped to see what she was doing and then to admire the mushrooms. She said it turned into a very fun and social moment, and suddenly she realized that without all the rain, she would not have experienced that moment.
>
> We encourage you to practice reframing as a class activity. One student can present a situation, and the others can come up with a reframe. Or you can generate a list of situations and ask students to try their hand at reframing. Inevitably, students will bring up tragic events such as natural disasters and global pandemics. But just as inevitably, communities learn from these events, rally around each other, and develop creative solutions, alternatives, or preventatives.

Activity 3-3: Gratitude Practice

A growing body of research finds that a simple gratitude practice can improve well-being among nurses and other healthcare workers (Sexton & Adair, 2019). Commit to taking time at the end of each day to write down three good things that happened to you during the day. These can be exciting events such as acing an exam or receiving a job offer, but most likely, they will be more humble moments. You might appreciate a delicious meal, an unexpected connection with a friend, a nap, or a sunny day.

You may choose to write your three good things in a small notebook, on your phone, or on your laptop. The most important thing is to do it regularly for at least 10 days. You will begin to notice that throughout the day, your attention and thoughts will be drawn toward those good things around you and away from those things that produce negative feelings.

If you would like to take this exercise a step further, pick one good thing each day and reflect on the people and events that made that good thing possible. For example, if you are grateful for a hot cup of coffee, think about the barista who made it to work that day and the workers who manufactured the cups; you will increase your sense of connection with the world around you.

> Here are two resources that you might want to share in class:
>
> **A. J. Jacobs TED Talk:**
> https://www.ted.com/talks/a_j_jacobs_my_journey_to_thank_all_the_people_responsible_for_my_morning_coffee
>
> **365 Grateful Project:**
> https://www.youtube.com/watch?v=AedIvmd8MJA
> Website: https://365grateful.com

Activity 3-4: Positivity Portfolio

A *positivity portfolio* is a collection of objects, words, or photos that stirs positive emotions in the viewer or reader. Positivity portfolios are more common than we realize. A collection of photos, plants, and seashells on someone's desk is a positivity portfolio. Refrigerator magnets that remind a family of their travels together is a positivity portfolio. A collection of favorite quotes and a laptop or water bottle covered in stickers are positivity portfolios. A playlist can be a positivity portfolio. Create your own portfolio in any way you choose. All that matters is that you create a collection of items that make you feel a positive emotion, such as happiness, contentment, or peace.

> Ask students to spend the week looking for positivity portfolios or ask where they have seen some in the past: desktops filled with family photos, laptops with stickers, dorm doors and walls, Pinterest boards, collections, pins on jackets and backpacks, and so on.

Activity 3-5: Vision Board

We move toward the image of the future that we hold in our heads, and the more positive that vision, the more positive our future. Remember the story of Ryan Speedo Green, the young man who saw his first opera at the Met and visualized himself performing at that same stage someday. Creating positive visions of our future is a remarkably powerful tool.

To create a vision board, gather a stack of old magazines, scissors, a piece of cardstock or cardboard, and a glue stick. Give yourself at least an hour (set a timer) to flip through the magazines and cut out photos and words that represent the future you are seeking. Relax. What dreams do you have for yourself? (This exercise can be done for the upcoming year or a longer time frame, whichever seems best to you.) Cut and glue the pictures to your cardstock and keep the collage somewhere you can see it regularly.

> Depending on your time limitations and class size, this is a wonderful activity to do in groups. It is relaxing to sit and flip through magazines and cut and paste, quietly, beside friends or peers. We encourage you to ask students to share their completed vision boards and talk a little about their future goals and dreams.

Activity 3-6: Vision Board, With No Glue

Are you trying to make a difficult decision about your future? Is there something you desire, but you are having trouble achieving it? Create a quiet space and give yourself at least a half hour to do this activity. Visualize your life one year from now. What does it look like? The power is in the details. Imagine yourself waking up in the morning. Where are you? What do you eat for breakfast? Is someone with you, or are you alone? Go through your entire day in this future life, focusing on your work, your friends, the activities of your day. *Remember—details, details, details.* Pay attention to how you feel. On a piece of paper, write down as many details as you can remember.

reflect & journal

- We hope this chapter gave you a lot of ideas and food for thought. Which activities were the most helpful? Were any so compelling that you think you could include them in your self-care toolkit?
- "Our focus is our fate." Spend a few moments writing about your own focus and how it affects your well-being in the short and long term.

references

Baumeister, R. F., Bratslavsky, E., Finkenauer, C., & Vohs, K. D. (2001). Bad is stronger than good. *Review of General Psychology, 5*(4), 323–370. https://doi.org/10.1037/1089-2680.5.4.323

Haizlip, J., May, N., Schorling, J., Williams, A., & Plews-Ogan, M. (2012). The negativity bias, medical education, and the culture of academic medicine: Why culture change is hard. *Academic Medicine, 87*(9), 1205–1209. https://doi.org/10.1097/ACM.0b013e3182628f03

Sexton, J. B., & Adair, K. C. (2019). Forty-five good things: A prospective pilot study of the Three Good Things well-being intervention in the USA for healthcare worker emotional exhaustion, depression, work-life balance and happiness. *BMJ Open, 9*(3), e022695. https://doi.org/10.1136/bmjopen-2018-022695

Vaish, A., Grossmann, T., & Woodward, A. (2008). Not all emotions are created equal: The negativity bias in social-emotional development. *Psychological Bulletin, 134*, 383–403. https://doi.org/10.1037/0033-2909.134.3.383

Whitney, D., & Trosten-Bloom, A. (2003). *The power of appreciative inquiry: A practical guide to positive change*. Berrett-Koehler Publishers, Inc.

section II
The Mind of a Nurse

4
Self-Care, Communal Care, and Resilience Among Underrepresented Minoritized Nursing Professionals and Students

—Ebru Çayir

what

Read Chapter 4.

- Describe at least five unique challenges underrepresented minority (URM) nurses face.

  > The unique workplace stressors they face due to longstanding social and structural inequities—such as institutional and interpersonal racism, discrimination, and stereotyping—often remain invisible and unaddressed.
  >
  > - Daily exposure to racism—institutional discrimination, interpersonal racism
  > - Microaggressions
  > - Racial disparities that reduce URM retention in the nursing workforce
  > - The need to code switch in school and work, which takes an emotional toll
  > - Social exclusion
  > - Racialized experiences of emotional labor, negatively affecting self-care and care for patients
  >
  > Internationally educated nurses face institutional discrimination, inadequate acknowledgment and underuse of their expertise and previous work experience, lack of understanding and ignorance about their sociocultural background, and communication difficulties with their colleagues and patients (Ghazal et al., 2020; Xiao et al., 2014).

- The author states, "Nurses' experiences of emotional labor are not only gendered but also racialized." Explain what she means by this.

  > **Care is gendered.** Within the prevalent social structures of the US healthcare system, which are male-dominated, paternalistic, and hierarchical, emotional labor and provision of compassionate care mostly fall on the shoulders of female healthcare providers, particularly nurses (Bell et al., 2014; Erickson & Grove, 2008). The traditional image of a nurse is a woman who is capable of and enjoys providing tender care.
  >
  > **Nurses of color engage in "emotional double shift"** (Evans, 2013, p. 12) due to navigating everyday racial microaggressions and facing negative stereotype threat. Nurses' experiences of emotional labor are not only gendered but also racialized. Another challenge URM nurses may face is having to engage in a disproportionate amount of emotional labor when they care for patients (Cottingham et al., 2018). Systems of power and domination, including but not limited to racism, sexism, and class inequalities, mutually interact with one another to shape the ways in which practices of emotional labor are distributed disproportionately among nurses of different social locations. Race-related emotional experiences (e.g., facing microaggressions, stereotype threat), on top

of daily work stressors, exhaust URM nurses' emotional capital and in turn negatively affect their ability to engage in self-care and care for their patients (Cottingham et al., 2018).

- What unique barriers to self-care do URM nurses face?

In addition to all the barriers nurses face that were identified in Chapter 1, URM nursing students and professionals may experience significant stressors other than those related to the medical tasks they perform, such as institutional discrimination, racism, and microaggressions perpetrated by teachers, coworkers, or patients, which cause exclusion from the social fabric of the organization and lack of access to power (Griffith et al., 2007).

URM nurses are often underrepresented in management positions, thus lacking the resources and social networks that are necessary to influence organizational structures and practices (Griffith et al., 2007).

why

Why is communal care a potentially more effective strategy for well-being than self-care?

For the nursing community, *communal care* is a collective practice through which nurses can develop a multitude of strategies to care for each community member's well-being by mobilizing not only the individual but also interpersonal, organizational, and systems-level resources in reciprocal ways. This approach to cultivating health and wellness engages all constituents of a community, highlighting the interdependence between them and holding them responsible for each other's well-being. Communal care also acknowledges the diversity of health and wellness needs among nurses, aiming to create space for diverse, equitable, and inclusive approaches to addressing the problems of the most vulnerable members in the nursing community.

Wever and Zell (2017) argued that when individual self-care is proposed as "an antidote" for the negative impacts of the work within human service organizations, it "places the responsibility of managing the effects of social, cultural and organizational injustices squarely on the individual worker" (p. 210). Without ignoring the necessity for each advocate (or nurse, in our case) to be cognizant of their own well-being needs and to be proactive, they called for "a movement of caring for and acknowledging each other in human service organizations" (Wever & Zell, 2017, p. 211).

Students might want to consider the benefits of communal care for *all* nurses, not just URM nurses. What would a culture of communal care look like in a nursing work environment?

do

Activity 4-1: Responding to Discriminatory Behavior: Individuals

Have you experienced or observed racial or ethnic identity-based discriminative experiences during your training? If so, what was your response or the response of others? If possible, gather in a group of four to five peers, establish expectations for students to safely share their experiences, and begin this conversation. Give yourselves time to make sure that all voices are heard.

Activity 4-2: Responding to Discriminatory Behavior: Healthcare Institutions

Reflect on and discuss with your peers how healthcare institutions can address the issues URM nursing professionals and students experience. What types of resources are available in your institution that might help address these issues? Are there any structural and policy changes you would like to see?

Generate a list of policy and health system changes your team envisions that would build equity, inclusion, and diversity into your school or workplace.

reflect & journal

- Think about examples of communal care in your own life and how they have had an impact on your well-being. Now consider ways that communal care and similar well-being benefits can be cultivated in healthcare organizations. What would our healthcare organizations look like, and in what ways would they focus on diversity, inclusion, and equity?

- Dr. Çayir selected this quote by Maya Angelou to open her chapter: "My mission in life is not merely to survive, but to thrive; and to do so with some passion, some compassion, some humor, and some style." Imagine yourself in your role as a nurse. In what ways will you embody these qualities—passion, compassion, humor, and style—in your work and life?

references

Bell, A. V., Michalec, B., & Arenson, C. (2014). The (stalled) progress of interprofessional collaboration: The role of gender. *Journal of Interprofessional Care, 28*(2), 98–102. https://doi.org/10.3109/13561820.2013.851073

Cottingham, M. D., Johnson, A. H., & Erickson, R. J. (2018). "I can never be too comfortable": Race, gender, and emotion at the hospital bedside. *Qualitative Health Research, 28*(1), 145–158. https://doi.org/10.1177/1049732317737980

Erickson, R. J., & Grove, W. J. C. (2008). Emotional labor and health care. *Sociology Compass, 2*(2), 704–733. https://doi.org/10.1111/j.1751-9020.2007.00084.x

Evans, L. (2013). *Cabin pressure: African American pilots, flight attendants, and emotional labor.* Rowman & Littlefield.

Ghazal, L. V., Ma, C., Djukic, M., & Squires, A. (2020). Transition-to-U.S. practice experiences of internationally educated nurses: An integrative review. *Western Journal of Nursing Research, 42*(5), 373–392. https://doi.org/10.1177/0193945919860855

Griffith, D. M., Childs, E. L., Eng, E., & Jeffries, V. (2007). Racism in organizations: The case of a county public health department. *Journal of Community Psychology, 35*(3), 287–302. https://doi.org/10.1002/jcop.20149

Wever, C., & Zell, S. (2017). Re-working self-care: From individual to collective responsibility through a critical ethics of care. In B. Pease, A. Vreugdenhil, & S. Stanford (Eds.), *Critical ethics of care in social work: Transforming the politics and practices of caring* (pp. 207). Routledge.

Xiao, L. D., Willis, E., & Jeffers, L. (2014). Factors affecting the integration of immigrant nurses into the nursing workforce: A double hermeneutic study. *International Journal of Nursing Studies, 51*(4), 640–653. https://doi.org/10.1016/j.ijnurstu.2013.08.005

5
Self-Care for LGBTQIA+ Nursing Students

–Kim Acquaviva

what

Read Chapter 5.

- List the additional stressors faced by LGBTQIA+ nursing students.

    - Family expectations
    - Social norms and assumptions
    - Legally sanctioned discrimination, hate, and violence

    For your reference, you might want to refer to this white paper on how to improve the learning climate in nursing and other health professions schools: https://healthdiversity.pitt.edu/sites/default/files/RecommendationsforEnhancingLGBTClimateinHealthProfessionalSchools.pdf

- Given these additional stressors, self-care strategies are vitally important for the LGBTQIA+ nursing student. Describe the four LGBTQIA+–specific self-care strategies that the author suggests in this chapter.

    1. **Explore "outness" in your own time and your own way:** Come out when you feel safe to do so. There is no "right" way to come out or to be an LGBTQIA+ person in nursing school.

    2. **Find a mentor who shares your identity/ies:** This mentor doesn't have to share your identity, but if they do, they will be able to help you navigate nursing school and anticipate what to expect after you graduate.

    3. **Seek out healthy ways of being in community with people:** Finding LGBTQIA+ people and being in community with them outside of school (and bars) can be scary but rewarding. Seek out an LGBTQIA+ group doing something you love, such as sports or a hobby.

    4. **Focus on what your body can do, not on who your body can attract:** You (and your body) are perfect exactly as they are. Care for your body as the vehicle that will carry you through your life.

why

This chapter opens with the famous quote by Audre Lorde: "Caring for myself is not self-indulgence, it is self-preservation, and that is an act of political warfare" (Lord, 1988, p. 205). Why is caring for oneself an act of political warfare?

> You might find some interesting food for thought in this brief essay by Rituparna Som:
>
> https://www.vice.com/en/article/nexbpz/is-self-care-an-act-of-political-warfare
>
> She writes, "When you're presenting your individual 'self' to a society that creates and supports homogeneity, then yes, self-care is a way to say that YOU matter. YOU are worthy. As an act of rebellion—that seems on point."
>
> She also quotes Evette Dionne, who wrote, "And so saying that I matter, that I come first, that what I need and what I want matters I think is a radical act because it goes against everything that we've been conditioned to believe."

do

Activity 5-1: The Importance of Being Seen

If you identify as LGBTQIA+, how did it feel reading a chapter that was written in a voice that was clearly speaking to you? Think of times in your life when you have felt seen. What specific behaviors on the part of others make you feel this way?

If you identify as heterosexual and cisgender, how did it feel reading a chapter that was written in a voice that was clearly speaking to someone other than you? In what ways did the author express her compassion and understanding for her readers? Think of times in your life when you have felt seen for who you truly are. What specific behaviors on the part of others make you feel this way?

reflect & journal

- In what ways can you be more intentional about helping others feel truly seen by you?
- Identity is complex—LGBTQIA+ nursing students aren't just LGBTQIA+. They hold other identities simultaneously: Black, Latinx, Indigenous/Native, Jewish, Christian, Muslim, atheist, first-generation college student, and so on. LGBTQIA+ nursing students may also be persons with disabilities or persons for whom English is the second language they learned.

- What identities do you hold? How do you care for each of those identities?

  > Encourage all students to think about the identities they hold: a nursing student identity, a daughter, a friend, a leader, the jock, the funny one. Each role has a different persona. Invite students to explore how they present themselves in each role and how comfortable and authentic they feel in each. We hope they will develop additional empathy for themselves and for their fellow students who embody complex identities.

reference

Lorde, A. (1988). *A burst of light: And other essays.* Courier Dover Publications.

6
Racial Trauma and Healing

–Arminda Perch

what

Read Chapter 6.

- Explain what defines a trauma or traumatic event.

  - Trauma is a terrible experience that when it happens to you fundamentally shifts the way you think about yourself, others, and the world. It can result from various experiences, including but not limited to accidents, physical or sexual assault, illness, medical procedures, loss of a loved one, bullying, family dysfunction, and discrimination. Traumatic events are often experienced as life-threatening—physically or existentially.

- What are some of the responses individuals have to trauma?

  - Trauma can cause individuals to feel strong yet also the very natural emotions of overwhelm, terror, fear, anger, and sadness. Trauma can generate thoughts such as "I'm not safe," "I'm not in control," or responses such as a "keyed up" nervous system and a raised level of vigilance and hyper awareness. It is also natural to experience these responses for weeks or longer following the traumatic event.

  - Some individuals have trauma responses that do not recover naturally. These responses are often described as feeling "stuck." Lack of recovery can lead to a myriad of enduring problems: self-blame, guilt, shame, anxiety, depression, panic, post-traumatic stress, a sense of hopelessness or powerlessness, insomnia, gut issues, social isolation, nightmares, flashbacks, and negative thoughts patterns. These problems can become unbearable, leading us to avoid or escape them (Resick et al., 2017). We often avoid in very sophisticated ways such as staying busy, rushing through tasks, evading people or specific situations, coming late to meetings, going numb (sometimes with the assistance of alcohol or drugs), outbursts of anger, suppressing thoughts, or attempting to control our surroundings. These responses may seem reasonable because they help us feel better in the short term; however, avoidance behaviors stand in the way of long-term recovery (Barlow et al., 2018; National Center for PTSD, 2022).

- What is vicarious trauma?

  - *Vicarious trauma* refers to the emotional and psychological impact that individuals may experience when indirectly exposed to the trauma of others. It can occur when we are empathetically involved in someone else's suffering over prolonged periods. As professional caregivers, nurses and other medical professionals indirectly experience a patient's trauma regularly. The same symptoms characterize vicarious trauma as directly experienced trauma (Kennedy & Booth, 2022).

- Explain race-based stress and trauma (RBST) and its impact on those who experience it.

    RBST, or racial trauma, is a terrible experience that involves direct or indirect exposure to various forms of racial discrimination and harm (Cénat, 2023). Racial trauma is experienced individually and collectively, and examples include microaggressions, racial bias, racially motivated workplace bullying, unwarranted police harassment or violence against people of color, lack of adequate medical care due to racial stereotypes, and lack of diversity in the workplace (Williams, 2022). Racial trauma can be the result of one horrifying event or a series of events and can include direct experiences, vicarious encounters, or ongoing collective experiences (Metzger, 2021). Everyday racial stressors are initially felt as an emotional sting. However, as experiences accumulate, the sting grows into a severe emotional injury that can develop and manifest as rage, internalized devaluation, appropriation of negative judgments, voicelessness, hyperfocus on survival, a sense of estrangement, overexerting our energies in the way we do our work, and exhaustion (Hardy, 2023; Jones et al., 2019). *Racial trauma* can also be described as "a traumatic form of interpersonal violence which can lacerate the spirit, scar the soul, and puncture the psyche" (Hardy, 2013, p. 25). This indicates that these experiences can deeply penetrate our human spirit.

- What are the three central tasks required for recovery of racial trauma? What does each entail?

    1. **Stabilization.** Stabilization is associated with reestablishing a sense of safety and emotional self-regulation. The first work of stabilization and safety is recognizing that something happened and accepting that "I felt something" when it happened. We do not have to judge our feelings, but we do need to acknowledge them. Not acknowledging our feelings leads us to invalidate ourselves and deepens the impact of the experience. Acknowledgment causes us to stop fighting against the reality of what happened and accept that it hurt, and it helps us to be willing to observe, learn, and make sense of our experiences of racism (Williams, 2022).

    2. **Healing.** Healing from racial trauma is not merely a reduction of symptoms. It involves a soul-level liberation from distorted and damaging views about our own identity and humanity that are a product of systemic and historical racism. When it comes to trauma work, we cannot change the fact that something has happened to us, but we can change the impact of what happened. We can think of healing as an ongoing detoxification process that removes or neutralizes toxins (i.e., impact of racial trauma) poisoning our system. These toxins can be generated internally or come from external sources. Detoxification can take place naturally, but when we have come to a place in our health where our symptoms are uncontrolled, we may need to make significant changes to how we think and live.

    3. **Empowerment.** Empowerment is a stage of growth and personal agency. It is a new season in which we are no longer encumbered by the weights that previously beset us. We can intentionally move through our experiences authentically. This does not mean that we no longer experience RBST, but we are now able to recover from it

> more quickly because we have the right tools for coping, resilience, and just living out our regular lives. It may have been a long and rough journey, but we know how to remind ourselves that we are worth the effort and use our skills to navigate the waves. We also know how to forgive ourselves, have meaningful connections, and give and receive emotional nourishment to each other.

why

What is the goal of recovery from racial trauma?

> It is important to "engage in the deep, inner work necessary to healing the impact of racial trauma" in order to "become more in control of how we respond to stressors and traumatic experiences."

do

Activity 6-1: Learn More About Racial Trauma and Healing

If you have not experienced racial trauma yourself, some of the material in this chapter may have been new to you. You could take this as an invitation to learn more about the experiences of your peers or co-workers. If you are reading this text in a course, ask if the minoritized students would be comfortable talking about their experiences with racial trauma. It is important to create a safe space for sharing these stories. Other students should listen respectfully and ask curious questions if appropriate. If this sharing isn't an option, there are countless books, movies, and podcasts that can help us learn more about the experiences of others in our communities.

What resources are available to students in your school who have experienced racial trauma?

> Most universities have resources available for students who experience racial trauma, and it will be helpful to all students to identify, or revisit, what these are. This is also an opportunity to talk about Employee Assistance Programs (EAPs) available in most hospitals so students can think ahead about where they might turn during their work life. We have found that most undergraduates are unaware of EAP programs and what they offer.

Activity 6-2: Use the Tools

In this chapter, the author offers many concrete steps an individual can take to move toward healing. They are presented in the context of racial trauma and healing. If you are someone who has experienced racial trauma, what steps might you take today to begin your healing journey?

If you have not personally experienced racial trauma, how might the steps be helpful in coping with challenges in your own life?

reflect & journal

How has reading this chapter shifted your perspective and changed how you might interact with your peers and future patients?

references

Barlow, D., Farchione, T., Sauer-Zavala, S., Murray Latin, H., Ellard, K., Bullis, J., Bentley, K., Boettcher, H., & Cassiello-Robbins, C. (2018). *Unified protocol for transdiagnostic treatment of emotional disorders.* Oxford University Press.

Cénat, J. M. (2023). Complex racial trauma: Evidence, theory, assessment, and treatment. *Perspectives on Psychological Science: A Journal of the Association for Psychological Science, 18*(3), 675–687. https://doi.org/10.1177/17456916221120428

Hardy, K. (2013). Healing the hidden wounds of racial trauma. *Reclaiming Children and Youth, 22*(1), 25–28. https://sfgov.org/juvprobation/sites/default/files/Documents/juvprobation/JPC_2014/Healing_the_Hidden_Wounds_of_Racial_Trauma.pdf

Hardy, K. (2023). *Racial trauma: Clinical strategies and techniques for healing invisible wounds.* W. W. Norton & Company, Inc.

Jones, S. C. T., Brooks, J. H., Milam, A. J., Barajas, C. B., LaVeist, T. A., Kane, E., & Furr-Holden, C. D. M. (2019). Racial discrimination, John Henryism coping, and behavioral health conditions among predominantly poor, urban African Americans: Implications for community-level opioid problems and mental health services. *Journal of Community Psychology, 47*(5), 1032–1042. https://doi.org/10.1002/jcop.22168

Kennedy, S., & Booth, R. (2022). Vicarious trauma in nursing professionals: A concept analysis. *Nursing Forum, 57*(5), 893–897. https://doi.org/10.1111/nuf.12734

Metzger, I. (2021). *The CARE Package for racial healing: Cultivating awareness & resilience through empowerment.* Strive Publishing.

National Center for PTSD. (2022, Sept. 22). *Anger and trauma.* https://www.ptsd.va.gov/understand/related/anger.asp

Resick, P. A., Monson, C. M., & Chard, K. M. (2017). *Cognitive processing therapy: A comprehensive manual.* The Guilford Press.

Williams, M. (2022, May 18). *The racial trauma treatment protocol: A 12-session CBT approach for therapists working with racial wounds* [Digital Seminar]. https://catalog.pesi.com/item/the-racial-trauma-treatment-protocol-12session-cbt-approach-therapists-working-racial-wounds-97282

7
Narrative Practices

–Tim Cunningham

what

Read Chapter 7.

- This chapter is about paying attention. How can narrative practices, and other activities that foster deep awareness, help you become a better clinician?

  > Narrative practices have the capacity to increase empathy and attention skills as well as broaden self-awareness.
  >
  > Narrative practices, reflective writing, and intellectual discourse have a common thread: the necessity of paying close attention. Research on narrative medicine for nurses and physicians suggests that engaging closely with the arts or literature (e.g., if you're examining a piece of literature, spending time looking deeply into writing style, theme, tone, and voice) can, over time, increase empathy scores and attention scores on various scales (Mangione et al., 2018; Ward et al., 2012).
  >
  > Uniquely ours, lived experience is an important aspect of our lives to examine because from it, we will know ourselves better. In knowing ourselves better, we'll better understand our own critical self-care needs.

- Describe the three levels of resonance, or caring: sympathetic, empathetic, and compassionate.

  > *Sympathetic resonance* is an example of physical entrainment, in which periodic behavior of one object can be communicated to another, even when there are no direct physical connections between the two (Dawson & Meddler, n.d.). Sympathetic resonance is best observed in nonliving objects, like the strings of a violin or other musical instrument. *Empathetic resonance* is essentially connecting with—or vibrating with (if that's a phrase you can relate to)—another person's emotional state. Empathetic resonance is absolutely crucial when it comes to the healing arts, regardless of your profession within healthcare (Richards, 2018). As nurses, we experience empathetic resonance when we encounter a patient who is suffering. Through narrative practices that we'll explore in this chapter, you can practice your skills at empathetic resonance and reading "the space in between." It is in this "space in between" where the empathetic resonance passes and occurs.
  >
  > *Compassionate resonance* occurs when we recognize and connect with someone else's suffering and then take the next step of doing something about it. Compassion reflects action. It does not always mean that we will end the suffering of another, but we must make efforts (even if those efforts are thoughts) to help decrease it.

why

In considering our ability to reflect, refract, and deflect emotions, why is awareness of this phenomenon so important to nurses? What examples can you provide?

> When we feel emotions that others see and share, that is *reflection*; think, "Laughter is contagious." When others see us respond with an emotion and they respond in a different way, that is *refraction*. When others see us experiencing emotion and then shut down or display a flat affect, that is *deflection*. For nurses, it is important for us to be aware that patients, families, and even colleagues may be refracting or deflecting difficult emotions when they don't respond the way we might expect to respond. A mother whose child is gravely ill might not respond with tears, as we might expect. Instead, she might respond with stoicism or nervousness. It does not mean her concern isn't deep, but she may be deflecting or refracting her emotions.

do

Activity 7-1: Visual Arts

In groups of three or four, collectively select a famous painting or sculpture. You may consider browsing websites of a local art museum to find images on the web. Once you find the image, designate one person in the group to prompt discussion questions about the image. (This exercise may certainly be done on your own, but it is an excellent group activity.) Here is a list of museum websites:

- **The Tate Modern:** https://www.tate.org.uk
- **The Metropolitan Museum of Art:** https://www.metmuseum.org
- **Museo Botero:** https://www.banrepcultural.org/bogota/museo-botero
- **The National Bardo Museum:** http://www.bardomuseum.tn
- **Tokyo National Museum:** https://www.tnm.jp/?lang=en
- **National Museum Australia:** https://www.nma.gov.au

Ask the following questions of the group, and allow time for everyone to respond.

1. What comes to mind first when you see this image?
2. What is the first feeling (if any) that comes up for you?
3. Look closely now at the textures of the image. What do you see?

4. Look closely now at the colors in the image. What do you see?
5. What do you think the artist was trying to say with this piece of work?
6. If you could meet the artist right now, what would you tell them about this work?

> Activity 7-1 could be done as a classroom activity, as could reading Dr. Mathieu's poem together as a class. Or you might want to try the same activity with music. As a class, listen to Handel's "Largo from Xerxes: Ombra mai fu" or any other piece or genre.
>
> Music (allow at least 30 minutes to complete this exercise): In groups of three or four, listen to the selected piece at least three times, with your eyes closed, and let your mind wander to wherever it chooses to go. Designate one person in the group to prompt discussion questions about the music.
>
> Ask the following questions of the group and allow time for everyone, including the person giving the prompts, to respond.
>
> 1. What comes to mind first when you first listen to this music?
> 2. What is the first feeling (if any) that comes up for you?
> 3. Listen closely to the rhythm of the music. What do you hear?
> 4. Listen closely to the tone or mood that this music evokes. What do you hear?
> 5. What do you think the artist was trying to say with this piece of work?
> 6. If you could meet the artist right now, what would you tell them about this work?

Activity 7-2: Capturing Your Own Experience in Art

Think of a patient encounter or healthcare experience that had meaning to you. Select an art form—prose or poetry writing, painting, drawing, collage, music, photography—and convey your experience of this encounter. Relax and enjoy this process. There is no right or wrong, good or bad.

reflect & journal

- In this chapter, the author writes, "That calling [to become a nurse] is at the core of our lived experience. Uniquely ours, lived experience is an important aspect of our lives to examine because, from it, we will know ourselves better. In knowing ourselves better, we'll better understand our own individual and critical self-care needs." Write about your calling to become a nurse. What is your story?

- Select a narrative of health, illness, or healing to read. You may choose one of the books included in this chapter (e.g., *Violation*, *When Breath Becomes Air*, *Fun Home*) or choose one of the many others that have been written. If an entire book feels daunting, select an essay or short story. Use the narrative practice skills we have discussed to reflect on the work you chose. How did the work make you feel? How did it change you? What did it convey about the author and their experience of health, illness, or healing?

> **55-word stories.** We also refer you to Colleen Fogarty's (2010) work using "Fifty-Five Word Stories" for personal reflection and teaching. These are "brief pieces of creative writing that use elements of poetry, prose, or both to encapsulate key experiences in healthcare" (p. 400).
>
> Fogarty, C. T. (2010). Fifty-five word stories: "Small jewels" for personal reflection and teaching. *Family Medicine, 42*(6), 400–402. PMID: 20526906.

references

Dawson, M., & Meddler, D. (n.d.). *Dictionary of cognitive science*. University of Alberta. http://www.bcp.psych.ualberta.ca/~mike/Pearl_Street/Dictionary/contents/S/sympres.html

Mangione, S., Chakraborti, C., Staltari, G., Harrison, R., Tunkel, A. R., Liou, K. T., Cerceo, E., Voeller, M., Bedwell, W. L., Fletcher, K., & Kahn, M. J. (2018). Medical students' exposure to the humanities correlates with positive personal qualities and reduced burnout: A multi-institutional U.S. survey. *Journal of General Internal Medicine, 33*(5), 628–634. https://doi.org/10.1007/s11606-017-4275-8

Richards, R. (2018). Empathy and relational creativity. In R. Richards (Ed.), *Everyday creativity and the healthy mind* (pp. 243–265). Palgrave Macmillan.

Ward, J., Cody, J., Schaal, M., & Hojat, M. (2012). The empathy enigma: An empirical study of decline in empathy among undergraduate nursing students. *Journal of Professional Nursing, 28*(1), 34–40. https://doi.org/10.1016/j.profnurs.2011.10.007

8
Self-Care and Systemic Change: What You Need to Know

–Ashley Hurst

what

Read Chapter 8.

- There are pitfalls to focusing on individual self-care above all else. What are the author's concerns about this?

> Self-care practices alone do not ensure your well-being and professional satisfaction.
>
> The top causes of nursing burnout are excessive workload; moral distress; and lack of resources, professional autonomy, and decision-making authority (Mudallal et al., 2017).
>
> Self-care practices focus on the individual practitioner in isolation, rather than as a professional member of a team and complex system. One unintended consequence of promoting self-care practices as a way to reduce burnout is the focus on the individual practitioner as the problem to be fixed and not the systems causing the stressful work environment. Many hospitals and clinical practices offer programs that focus on the individual clinician, such as mindfulness-focused workshops and incentivized exercise programs. It follows, however, that if work stress is the result of inadequate staffing, lack of practice autonomy, and interprofessional collaboration, for example, self-care alone will not remedy these issues. Organizational leadership must focus on solving these complex issues with more than clinician-focused programs (NASEM, 2019; Shanafelt & Noseworthy, 2017).

- Explain moral distress in your own words. Provide at least one example.

> A leading cause of burnout in nurses is moral distress (Epstein et al., 2019). *Moral distress* is generally defined as the belief that you know the morally right thing to do but cannot do it because of external or internal barriers. The root causes of moral distress are institutional causes, not personal ones.
>
> Common causes of moral distress include continuing aggressive care not in the best interests of the patient; watching patient care suffer from lack of provider continuity; staffing shortages that endanger patient care; and poor team communication (Whitehead et al., 2015). However, moral distress is *experienced by* the individual nurse, physician, or other clinician. In other words, you experience moral distress, but its cause is rooted in the work environment.

- What is the #selfcare movement? Why is it potentially harmful for true well-being?

> The #selfcare social media movement is frequently presented as a hyper-feminine form of self-indulgence. From bubble baths to spa days, what is depicted on social media is

often a caricature of self-care practices aimed at selling products and competing with one's Instagram followers. The explosion of the #selfcare movement has created a $10-billion industry (Silva, 2017).

The #selfcare movement is often misleading and needs to be differentiated from the self-care practices in this book.

The #selfcare message echoes unhelpful gender stereotypes of pampered women and in no way reflects the mental work intrinsic to a true self-care practice.

Additionally, studies show that #selfcare is creating yet another arena for public display and competition, contributing to a negative self-image in those judging themselves lacking in Instagrammable self-care practices (Lieberman, 2018).

why

- Why is the "mythology of heroic, self-sacrificing women who cared for the sick" problematic for the well-being of today's nurses?

    Florence Nightingale's archetype of "the good nurse" may have lead to unfair and unjust expectations. The author writes, "We trust nurses to care for us and our loved ones, but it seems that we also trust them to bounce back from whatever adversity comes their way. Is this a fair and just expectation? Do we need nurses to be even more resilient so they can face even more trauma and distress? Or do we owe nurses meaningful change that reduces the traumatic and distressing situations they face in practice? Building nurses' personal resilience is certainly important. However, if the primary goal is their well-being, we must not ignore the underlying systemic issues that, if addressed, will reduce the distress and traumatic experiences nurses routinely face" (Barton et al., 2022).

do

Activity 8-1: The Mythology of Nursing

This chapter links the origin myths and stereotypes of nursing to many of the underlying systemic issues in healthcare today. Dig a little deeper into this notion of potentially harmful perceptions of nursing and nurses. What misperceptions have you personally encountered? What stereotypes did you grow up with? Have these stereotypical images changed since you've become a nursing student?

Activity 8-2: #selfcare

In Chapter 1, we invited you to do a Google search of self-care practices. Our goal was to give you a broad sense of the self-care activities and options available to you as you begin this journey. We suggested that you view your search results through a personal lens: What practices were appealing to you? Which were you curious to learn more about? Now we invite you to revisit your Google search, or do another one, and look at the search results through the #selfcare lens. Which create unrealistic expectations? Which may not be based in good science? Which promote unhelpful stereotypes? Which are actually ridiculous? Which might be harmful?

reflect & journal

- Imagine yourself in an unhealthy work environment. (We hope this doesn't happen to you.) What would you do in that situation? What options might you have?

- It is discouraging to think that your workplace may not prioritize the well-being of its employees. As we wrote in the editors' introduction to the textbook chapter, there is a tension between self-care and institutional responsibility. Give yourself some time and space to reflect and write on this difficult issue.

references

Barton, M., Kahn, B., Maitlis, S., & Sutcliffe, K. (2022, April 4). Stop framing wellness programs around self-care. *Harvard Business Review*. https://hbr.org/2022/04/stop-framing-wellness-programs-around-self-care

Epstein, E. G., Whitehead, P. B., Prompahakul, C., Thacker, L. R., & Hamric, A. B. (2019). Enhancing understanding of moral distress: The measure of moral distress for health care professionals. *AJOB Empirical Bioethics, 10*(2), 113–124. https://doi.org/10.1080/23294515.2019.1586008

Lieberman, C. (2018, Aug. 10). How self-care became so much work. *Harvard Business Review*. https://hbr.org/2018/08/how-self-care-became-so-much-work

Mudallal, R. H., Othman, W. M., & Al Hassan, N. F. (2017). Nurses' burnout: The influence of leader empowering behaviors, work conditions, and demographic traits. *Inquiry: A Journal of Medical Care Organization, Provision, and Financing, 54*. https://doi.org/10.1177/0046958017724944

National Academies of Sciences, Engineering, and Medicine. (2019). *Taking action against clinician burnout: A systems approach to professional well being*. The National Academies Press. https://doi.org/10.17226/25521

Shanafelt, T. D., & Noseworthy, J. H. (2017). Executive leadership and physician well-being: Nine organizational strategies to promote engagement and reduce burnout. *Mayo Clinic Proceedings, 92*(1), 129–146. https://www.mayoclinicproceedings.org/article/S0025-6196(16)30625-5/pdf

Silva, C. (2017, June 4). The millennial obsession with self-care. *NPR*. https://www.npr.org/2017/06/04/531051473/the-millennial-obsession-with-self-care

Whitehead, P. B., Herbertson, R. K., Hamric, A. B., Epstein, E. G., & Fisher, J. M. (2015). Moral distress among healthcare professionals: Report of an institution-wide survey. *Journal of Nursing Scholarship, 47*(2), 117–125. https://doi.org/10.1111/jnu.12115

9

Strengths-Based Self-Care: Good Enough, Strong Enough, Wise Enough

—Tim Cunningham

what

Read Chapter 9.

- What is the "victim narrative"? How can it be detrimental to well-being?

   > The "victim narrative" is a response to adversity that blames others rather than taking responsibility; in other words, it's allowing yourself to believe that you are stymied by factors far beyond your control, and worse, that you can just give up because of them (Edwards et al., 2010).
   >
   > The victim narrative can lead to withdrawal, pulling away from social connections, and giving up. The "victim" feels powerless to make change, and that feeling becomes a self-fulfilling prophecy.

- Explain posttraumatic growth (PTG) in your own words.

   > In essence, PTG encourages people to consider what they have learned from past traumatic experiences, how they have grown emotionally, and how have they become psychologically stronger after stressful or traumatic experiences.

- What are the five elements of PTG?

   1. **Personal strength:** How do you see yourself as changed because of the traumas you've experienced, and how have you become stronger because of them?
   2. **Closer relationships:** When you think about the relationships that have withstood the traumas in your life, how have they changed? Which ones have lasted, and what strength do you find in them?
   3. **Greater appreciation for life:** How do you see life differently now as a result of your traumas? What do you value more now? What in life brings you joy?
   4. **New possibilities:** Do you think about certain aspects of your life differently now, and in doing so, how have those perspective changes inspired you to experience innovative ideas? What do you do differently now in your life that builds resilience for yourself and others?
   5. **Spiritual development:** What are your new views on spirituality, having withstood the traumas in your life? How have these views changed, and what sort of spiritual wisdom have you noticed in your own self?

- List the five aspects of high emotional intelligence.

   1. Self-awareness
   2. Self-regulation

3. Motivation
4. Empathy
5. Social skills

why

Why might "not taking it personally" be one of the most valuable tools in your self-care toolkit?

> This exercise provides another opportunity to help students consider different ways of responding to difficult patients and families. Patients come to us not on their best days, but often on their worst.

do

Activity 9-1: Growth From Trauma

Take some time to read about a person you admire. They could be a civil rights or political leader, community advocate, artist, scientist, businessperson, or celebrity. You might choose a nurse, friend, or loved one. As you learn about this person, consider any trauma that they experienced. How did that trauma lead to transformation and growth? What strengths did they draw on to help them navigate the traumatic event?

> You might want to share some of the videos that are available (and free) on the University of Virginia Wisdom through Adversity website. The site includes a 55-minute documentary, *Choosing Wisdom*, but there are also smaller clips, including an eight-minute video of Lawrence Calhoun explaining the history of posttraumatic growth (in the "For Physicians" section).
>
> https://med.virginia.edu/wisdom/about-our-work/pbs-documentary-book/

Activity 9-2: Inherent Strengths Inventory

This chapter contends that we all have inherent strengths, and we can build on these strengths as a form of self-care. In other words, we don't have to begin from scratch, and we don't have to learn everything anew. We each have qualities and characteristics that will help us navigate adversity, grow, and maintain our well-being. We invite you to create your own strengths inventory. Consider traits that are included in this chapter, but we encourage you to expand your view to include other qualities as well.

reflect & journal

How have you moved through adversity or trauma in your life? How did that experience transform you in good ways and bad?

reference

Edwards, D., Burnard, P., Bennett, K., & Hebden, U. (2010). A longitudinal study of stress and self-esteem in student nurses. *Nurse Education Today, 30*(1), 78–84. https://doi.org/10.1016/j.nedt.2009.06.008

section III
The Body and Spirit of a Nurse

10
Reclaiming, Recalling, and Remembering: Spirituality and Self-Care

—Robin Brown-Haithco

what

Read Chapter 10.

- How does this author define "spirituality"?

  > For the purposes of this chapter, *spirituality* is that which sustains and nurtures us in the critical, chaotic, suffering moments in our lives. It is not necessarily related to (but certainly could be) any particular religious belief or theological understanding. It is defined by those things that give us meaning in life, the core beliefs and values that ground and center us, and the relationships that we trust and depend on to hold us when we can no longer hold ourselves. It is what invites us to find joy in the midst of sorrow and sadness, and it is what allows us to move toward gratitude and hope when what we love most is about to slip away from us.

- What does the author mean by "vocation"?

  > *Vocation* is a voice calling from within inviting us to do that which brings us joy while meeting the deepest needs of those in the world (Buechner, 1993, p. 119). I fully believe that our vocation calls us, and when we listen deeply to our heart's desires, we will respond to that call with excitement and passion. When what we do matches the joy and passion within us, whatever bumps in the road we may encounter will not deter us from our commitment and purpose in life.

- Describe the term "paradoxical thinking" and give three examples.

  > The author writes, "I have learned in my work with clinicians that the work of healthcare is becoming more and more stressful. Patients seem to be arriving sicker and sicker, and families are arriving with heightened emotions that often get directed toward the staff who are caring for their loved ones. Some staff are able to go beneath the surface emotion (often anger) and see the deeper emotion (fear of losing their loved one). When this translation of the surface emotion occurs, staff are able to live in the tension between the two. This is what I mean by *paradoxical thinking*—holding two contradictory thoughts or opinions or emotions simultaneously—living in the tension of the both/and. The family is angry and afraid at the same time. The emotion most easily recognized is the anger; the one that can go unnoticed is the fear, the emotion that makes us more vulnerable."
  >
  > Examples include anger and fear; anxiety and excitement; grief and relief.
  >
  > This provides another opportunity to talk about fostering compassion and "not taking it personally," as discussed in Chapter 9.

why

Why is it important to acknowledge and talk about "our true selves"?

> Our task throughout life is to recall the "true self" given to us at birth. It is this recalling that will invite us to live fully into our gifts and reclaim our health and wholeness. The author suggests that living into our true selves will support our own well-being as well as our ability to care for others with compassion.

do

Activity 10-1: Defining a Belief System

Consider your own belief system, or your guiding principles, and write answers to the following questions.

- Who, or what, encouraged you to believe as you do? What in your own life narrative has led you to these beliefs?
- Are your beliefs based on a traditional spiritual practice or something else?
- What specifically are your guiding principles?
- How do your guiding principles affect your daily living? (This could include decision-making, self-care, or simply the way you show up in the world.)
- How do you nurture your spiritual practice or belief system?
- Tell a story about a time that your spiritual practice allowed you to move through a challenging time to a place of peace, compassion, love, or hope.

reflect & journal

- How will your values or beliefs guide your professional role as a nurse?
- The author includes a quote by Parker Palmer (2020) who says we will find our vocation by accepting the "treasure of true self" we already possess. He encourages us to listen for and nurture that true self. Do you think you know who your true self is?

references

Buechner, F. (1993). *Wishful thinking*. HarperOne.
Palmer, P. (2000). *Let your life speak*. Jossey-Bass.

11
Sleep, Exercise, and Nutrition: Self-Care the Kaizen Way

–Tim Cunningham

what

Read Chapter 11.

- Explain the philosophy of Kaizen. How does it relate to a self-care practice?

  > *Kaizen* is a Japanese term that means "good change." Car manufacturing companies, like Toyota, have used this concept to identify small problems and feasible changes that can be made to fix them (Hosono, 2020). By taking a "bite-sized" approach to change, rather than trying to fix and change everything at once, change can happen, sustainably, over time. What's best about Kaizen is that change is manageable. You don't have to climb the mountain today or finish the whole marathon right away—you just have to take one step forward. When you think of Kaizen, think about incremental change and remember that self-care is a practice. It needs repetition, and it can become easier over time.

- List five nonpharmacological sleep aids.

  - Follow regular sleep cycles, when possible.
  - Make sure your bedroom is quiet, dark, relaxing, and at a comfortable temperature.
  - Remove electronic devices, such as TVs, computers, and smartphones, from the bedroom.
  - Avoid large meals, caffeine, and alcohol before bedtime.
  - Get some exercise. Being physically active during the day can help you fall asleep more easily at night.
  - Limit your caffeine intake during the day.
  - Avoid exercise late in the day.
  - Don't smoke.
  - Take a hot bath or shower before bed.
  - Keep your bedroom cool.
  - Turn the clock face away from your bed so you don't "watch the clock" when you're having trouble sleeping.
  - Try to get 30 minutes of natural sunlight each day.
  - Try aromatherapy.
  - Nap during the day.
  - Use sleep apps, such as Calm.
  - Try reading before bed.

- Relax your facial, neck, and shoulder muscles.
- Try "resourcing," as described in Chapter 4. Thinking about things that create positive or neutral feelings can slow down "rabbit brain" that prevents sleep.

• What are some of the well-being benefits of exercise? Of sexual activity?

- Sleep enhancer
- Physical health benefits: heart disease prevention, diabetes self-management, and so on
- Emotional and spiritual benefits
- Social connection

Sexual activity can buffer the stress of everyday life. In a study examining sexual habits, sex appeared to relieve stress by disrupting the escalation of stress from one day to the next (Ein-Dor & Hirschberger, 2012). Sex also produces health benefits, including maintaining circulator, neural, and muscular functionality of genitalia; acting as a preventive for prostate cancer in men; and counteracting vaginal atrophy in women (Levin, 2007). Further, sexual intimacy can foster the desire needed for durable relationships. Relationships are essential for coping throughout life, and they incur advantages.

• What are the barriers to healthy, nutritious eating faced by many nurses? (You may want to refer to Chapter 1 in the textbook as well.)

Barriers to nutritious eating include long work hours and exhaustion, making it difficult to prepare healthy meals. Nurses often work in unhealthy food cultures where baked goods and vending machines are plentiful but healthy options are not.

why

There are so many voices (experts and otherwise) telling us what to eat to maintain good health. In determining your own nutrition choices, who is the most important expert and why?

Listen to your body. It's as simple as that. Students will explore this concept more in Activities 11-1 and 11-2.

do

Activity 11-1: The Sleep-Exercise-Nutrition Triangle

This is an exercise to foster awareness of the connection between the three sides of the sleep-exercise-nutrition triangle and to help you pay attention to your own physical well-being. For seven days, keep track of your sleep, physical activity, and nutrition with simple +, –, or = signs. + indicates that you feel you did well in caring for yourself and meeting your physical needs; – indicates that you think you could have done better; and = indicates you aren't sure, or you are simply satisfied but not impressed. If you'd prefer, you may provide more detailed information in your chart, but our goal is to keep things simple.

Day	Sleep	Exercise	Nutrition	Notes
Example	+	–	=	Pouring rain; couldn't run Ate OK; didn't snack
1				
2				
3				
4				
5				
6				
7				

After seven days, can you see any patterns? If you had poor sleep on certain days, did exercise and nutrition suffer on those days, too? Are you consistently getting enough sleep but not enough exercise? Describe all the patterns that you notice. What factors had an impact on your physical self-care during this week?

Activity 11-2: Paying Attention

As you went through the week charting your physical self-care, we expect that you may have been paying close attention to your body in a new way. What kinds of things did you notice? What messages did your body send you? For example, how did your body feel after drinking beverages that contain sugar, caffeine, or alcohol?

Activity 11-3: The Kaizen Way

Consider what you learned this week using a Kaizen mindset. Where do you see opportunities for small steps that might result in change? Think about the sleep-exercise-nutrition triad, and identify one small change you can make. Commit to it for 10 days. We offer a few suggestions to get you thinking. Of course, refer to the *Self-Care* textbook and other sources for more ideas.

- Take the stairs instead of using the elevator.
- Turn off all screens 15 minutes before you lie down to sleep.
- Eat vegetarian for one meal a day.
- Pack healthy snacks—fruit, sugar-free yogurt, trail mix—in your backpack.
- Park farther away and walk.
- Use a sleep app to help you fall asleep.
- Eat one meal each day slowly and mindfully.
- Drink a glass of water first thing in the morning.

If this exercise resonates with you, consider adding one small change to the mix each week. Notice what larger changes begin to happen in your life.

reflect & journal

- What if, in this moment, you are good enough? We can say with surety that you are good enough. This chapter is not about being good or bad but about caring for yourself, especially your physical self. This chapter is about paying attention to your body so that you can respond to its needs. If your body needs something (more sleep, more movement, better fuel), you can make those changes slowly, one at a time.
- Write down all the reasons that you want to care for your body.

references

Ein-Dor, T., & Hirschberger, G. (2012). Sexual healing: Daily diary evidence that sex relieves stress for men and women in satisfying relationships. *Journal of Social and Personal Relationships, 29*(1), 126–139. https://doi.org/10.1177/0265407511431185

Hosono, A. (2020). Kaizen toward learning, transformation, and high-quality growth: Insights from outstanding experiences. In *Workers, managers, productivity* (pp. 45–67). Palgrave Macmillan, Singapore.

Levin, R. J. (2007). Sexual activity, health and well-being—The beneficial roles of coitus and masturbation. *Sexual and Relationship Therapy, 22*(1), 135–148. https://doi.org/10.1080/14681990601149197

12
Reflections on Self-Care and Your Clinical Practice

—Joy Miller

what

Read Chapter 12.

> This chapter will give your students a chance to visualize themselves fitting self-care practices into their daily work routines. None of the activities described require extra time or money; they are all done in the context of a nurse's busy day. This chapter also reinforces the belief that we all have the power to choose how we respond in any given situation.

- How does this author create in-the-moment self-care opportunities in the middle of a busy clinical practice?

  - Checking in with herself throughout the day: "How am I feeling?"
  - Using transition rituals
  - Honoring her own feelings, naming them, and writing them down
  - Journaling
  - Using "mini-moments" for gratitude reflections or deep breathing, recalling a happy memory
  - Making eye contact with others and expressing gratitude
  - Grounding (see also Chapter 4)
  - Deflecting and redirecting
  - Establishing and following her personal frame of reference
  - Practicing Tonglen
  - Establishing and maintaining boundaries

- What is a transition ritual?

> A *transition ritual* is an intentional opportunity to prepare for and decompress from work shifts. In some cases, it is also an opportunity to name and acknowledge feelings and emotions. The author writes, "When I first started working as a nurse, I realized I needed a transition ritual to start and end my shifts. My way to do this is through journaling. By writing, I honor and validate my feelings, and without judgment, I can move through the emotions I am experiencing at the start of my day. This allows me to be more focused on my patients and families. As I leave work, particularly after a long and stressful shift, I sometimes do the same thing. This provides a positive transition to being at home with my family."

- What does the author mean when she writes about "set an intention" or "intention setting"?

> She writes about this in the context of her Tonglen practice, and it describes her intentions about how she "shows up" for her patients. She writes, "When I practice Tonglen with my patients, I find the ability to connect to something tangible, something I could focus on when faced with any kind of suffering. Each person's definition of suffering is different, and we are all showing up to an encounter with our own struggles, successes, views, feelings, biases, and values. It is when we can find a generosity for another and offer them loving-kindness that we can transform how we show up. For example, when I am about to cross the threshold of a patient's room, I take three deep breaths. In those breaths I am receiving and giving loving-kindness before I even interact with the child and family in the room. I'm setting my intention from a foundation of kindness, in anticipation of what I will receive."

why

Why does the author sometimes cringe when she looks back on her early days as a nurse?

> The author writes, "I was not always self-aware, and I projected my feelings in a way that didn't serve me or my patients. In my desire to be helpful, I was certain I knew how someone felt and therefore, what they needed. I quickly came up with *my* truth about what they were experiencing, and even though I was well intentioned, I couldn't possibly know. I was serving my truth over theirs."

do

Activity 12-1: Transition Rituals

The chapter author uses journaling as a transition activity before and after her shifts. We know other nurses who use prayer, exercise, music, or meditation to help them prepare or decompress. Another rubs the leaves of a plant between her fingers when she walks past a garden on the way to her car. What transition rituals have you used in the past, even if you didn't name them as such? Try at least one transition ritual this week as you come and go to school or your clinical rotations.

Activity 12-2: To-Be-Joyful (*Not* a To-Do) List

In a chapter sidebar, Jennifer shares ways that she cares for herself on her days off. One way is to make a list of activities; the list makes her feel productive and allows her to intentionally focus on self-care. "This list keeps me reminded of activities outside of work that help me de-stress and stay organized. As I cross these tasks off my list, I earn my sense of productivity and feel ready to give back to others around me."

Imagine that you have all the time in the world to do things that make you happy. Write a list of these activities.

Activity 12-3: Frames of Reference

Review the author's description of her frames of reference, her guiding principles for showing up as a nurse. What frames of reference do you think would serve you well in your clinical practice? How do they build on the guiding principles that you live by today?

reflect & journal

- The self-care textbook focuses a lot of attention on physical self-awareness—noticing when you are tense, tired, thirsty, and more. This chapter approaches self-awareness from a different perspective. What kind of self-awareness makes the author the kind of nurse that she is?

- We especially love the author's description of Tonglen practice and how she uses the practice to foster loving-kindness toward those she encounters in her practice. We encourage you to learn more about this practice as a way to "set your intentions" toward your patients.

- The chapter author closes by writing about boundaries as a form of self-care. What are your boundaries in your life today? What additional boundaries would you like to establish?

section IV
The Transition to Nursing Practice

13
Supportive Professional Relationships: Nurse Residency Programs, Preceptors, and Mentors

–Carrie McDermott & Millie Sattler

what

Read Chapter 13.

- List the seven major challenges that newly licensed registered nurses face.

  1. Delegation
  2. Prioritization
  3. Managing care delivery
  4. Decision-making
  5. Collaboration
  6. Conflict resolution
  7. Self-confidence

  (Kramer et al., 2012).

- What are the goals of transition-to-practice nurse residency programs?

  A structured transition-to-practice nurse residency program (NRP) provides a means of social support and a rich resource for mentoring. These programs are designed to help new nurses adjust to the realities of the nursing profession, support development in the professional role, and provide guidance for self-care during the transition to practice and beyond (Fink et al., 2008; Goode et al., 2016).

- Describe the benefits of having a mentor.

  Mentoring can decrease stress levels in new graduate nurses and decrease anxiety in student nurses by providing socialization and emotional support (Kim et al., 2013; Van-Patten & Bartone, 2019).

  Student nurses have reported that mentoring has given them insight into the world of nursing, increased their confidence, increased their understanding of how to deal with difficult situations, and better prepared them for the realities of nursing (Lavoie-Tremblay et al., 2018).

- A nurse mentor can serve as a coach, counselor, confidant, encourager, friend, visionary, and resource. What roles should a mentor not embrace?

  Mentors should avoid embracing the roles of advocate, mediator, judge, boss, or magician.

why

Why should nurses and mentors set specific goals, and what might they entail?

> The goals you set with your mentor will provide a road map for where you want to go and how to get there. Goals could include the following:
> - Explore a particular career option
> - Establish a career direction
> - Ensure that you complete all the needed qualifications for the desired job
> - Decide on an academic program to pursue and begin enrollment
> - Improve working relationships with your supervisor and coworkers
> - Develop technical or professional skills in a growing area
> - Initiate and nurture a network of individuals who can help you in a newly identified career
>
> **Classroom activities:** We encourage you to lead a class discussion about effective mentors the students have had. What made them effective mentors?
>
> Share your own experience as a mentor and a mentee.
>
> Ask students to interview other faculty or preceptors about their mentoring experiences.

do

Activity 13-1: Investigate Nurse Residency Programs

Spend some time researching hospitals or health systems and their nurse residency programs (NRPs). Do they meet all the criteria outlined in this chapter, such as being nine to 12 months long, having an evidence-based curriculum, and so on? Are they accredited by the Commission on Collegiate Nursing Education or the American Nurses Credentialing Center? Do they offer evidence-based practice projects? (Review the NRP checklist at the end of the chapter.)

Activity 13-2: S.M.A.R.T. Goal Setting

Goal setting is an important part of the mentoring experience for both the mentee and the mentor. But what is a good goal? What are some criteria by which you can assess the strength of a goal? One way to structure goals is by using the S.M.A.R.T. goal approach. S.M.A.R.T. stands for Specific, Measurable, Achievable, Relevant, and Time-based. Consider one goal for yourself that you can achieve this month. It can be anything related to school, work, home, or self-care. In the following table, complete a S.M.A.R.T. diagram for your goal. Enter the name of your goal and generate the S.M.A.R.T. steps you will take to achieve it. Once you write this out, take steps toward completing that goal.

Name of Goal:	Responses:
Specific: Write out details about what this goal entails.	
Measurable: Write out exactly how you will measure accomplishment of this goal.	
Achievable: Is this goal achievable? How do you know? What have you achieved before this point that will help you know you can reach this one?	
Relevant: Write how this goal aligns with who you are, your personal beliefs, and your larger goals in life.	
Time-based: What is the realistic time frame during which you can begin to work on this goal and when you plan to achieve it? Are there milestones or checkpoints along the way that you can list to hit while you are achieving this goal?	

reflect & journal

- It's not all about the mentor. It is also the mentee's responsibility to collaborate effectively with the mentor and develop a trusting relationship. Zachary (2012) came up with nine essential mentee skills, listed next. Consider your own skills for each of these areas. Where are your strengths, and where might you need some improvement? What might you do to strengthen some of these skills?

    1. Ability to receive and give feedback
    2. Self-directed
    3. Open communicator
    4. Taking initiative
    5. Valuing self-reflection
    6. Ability to listen
    7. Ability to follow through
    8. Relationship building
    9. Ability to set goals

- In today's fast-paced "gig economy," some say that mentoring in nursing may be a dying art. How can you serve as a mentor to others today and in the future? Perhaps you are already serving in a mentoring role, either formal or informal. How can you reignite the art of mentoring?

references

Fink, R., Krugman, M., Casey, K., & Goode C. (2008, July-August). The graduate nurse experience: Qualitative residency program outcomes. *Journal of Nursing Administration, 38*(7–8), 341–348. https://doi.org/10.1097/01.NNA.0000323943.82016.48

Goode, C. J., Ponte, P. R., & Havens, D. S. (2016). Residency for transition into practice: An essential requirement for new graduates from basic RN programs. *Journal of Nursing Administration, 46*(2), 82–86. https://doi.org/10.1097/NNA.0000000000000300

Kim, S. C., Oliveri, D., Riingen, M., Taylor, B., & Rankin, L. (2013). Randomized controlled trial of graduate-to-undergraduate student mentoring program. *Journal of Professional Nursing, 29*(6), e43–e49. https://doi.org/10.1016/j.profnurs.2013.04.003

Kramer, M., Maguire, P., Halfer, D., Budin, W. C., Hall, D. S., Goodloe, L., Klaristenfeld, J., Teasley, S., Forsey, L., & Lemke, J. (2012). The organizational transformative power of nurse residency programs. *Nursing Administration Quarterly, 36*(2), 155–168. https://doi.org/10.1097/NAQ.0b013e318249fdaa

Lavoie-Tremblay, M., Sanzone, L., Primeau, G., & Lavigne, G. L. (2018). Group mentorship programme for graduating nursing students to facilitate their transition: A pilot study. *Journal of Nursing Management, 27*(1), 66–74. https://pubmed.ncbi.nlm.nih.gov/30198617/

Van Patten, R. R., & Bartone, A. S. (2019). The impact of mentorship, preceptors, and debriefing on the quality of program experiences. *Nurse Education in Practice, 35,* 63–68. https:/doi.org/10.1016/j.nepr.2019.01.007

14
Healthy Work Environment: How to Choose One for Your First Job

–Dorrie K. Fontaine

what

Read Chapter 14.

- List the six standards for establishing and sustaining a healthy work environment (HWE).

  1. Skilled communication
  2. True collaboration
  3. Effective decision-making
  4. Appropriate staffing
  5. Meaningful recognition
  6. Authentic leadership

  You may ask: What is your favorite standard, the one that resonates the most for you? Share your own ideas.

- "Skilled communication" is a broad standard that includes a range of important topics. List at least five aspects of skilled communication in an HWE.

  Aspects include developing proficiency in communicating with patients and families to build relationship-centered care, strengthen trust in patients and team members, and prevent miscommunication and errors in patient care.

  Foster respect and eliminate disrespect (follow ANA guidelines).

  Identify bullying behaviors and cite examples of subtle and overt ones.

- What distinguishes the Daisy Award as a meaningful form of recognition for nurses?

  The Daisy Award originated as one family's way to honor their son in his courageous battle with a rare blood disease and the nurses who cared for him. The Barnes family's passion and caring for the work of nurses has made this award a personal one for the nurse and hospital, as well as a national recognition. Nurses can be nominated by their peers, supervisors, and family members of a patient.

why

Why are some environments healthier than others? What factors have you observed in clinical settings that have led you to say, "This would be a good place to work," or, "This is not a place I would like to work"?

> In class discussions, ask for specific instances the student has witnessed and link back to one of the six standards, as in "good example of authentic leadership in that nurse manager's actions," or "sounds like the unit's nurses do not have a good way to communicate if this bullying is happening."
>
> This chapter is ripe for discussion opportunities. We have listed a few conversation starters here:
> - 100,000 hours in a full career: Can you find a way to visually display this remarkable number? Is it overwhelming for students to think about? (For you?)
> - Discussion of the nurse-physician relationship: What have students observed in their clinicals or in other settings?
> - Discussion of priorities in choosing a first job.
> - Meaningful recognition discussion: What kinds of recognition have your students observed? What kinds of recognition are most valuable to them? What do different types of recognition tell us about the nursing profession?
> - Anxieties about first jobs.
> - Discussion of HWE standards in the clinical environments where students have worked.

do

Activity 14-1: Identifying Priorities for Your First Job

Reflect on the priorities you might consider when choosing your first job in nursing. Rank the following seven criteria on level of importance from 1 to 7, where 1 has the highest importance to you and 7 has the lowest, at least in the early stages of your career. Use the table to rank these items and briefly describe your reasoning or considerations for each ranking. We have included additional rows for you to add other priorities, if needed.

> We encourage you to put yourself, as the instructor, in the students' shoes. How did you choose your first position? Was it a difficult choice? What factors did *you* consider? Continuous nursing shortages have made many openings available across the US. Is this making decisions easier or harder for your students?

Priority	Rank (1–7)	Reasons for Ranking/Factors to Consider
Geographic location		
Specialty		
Reputation of organization		
Proximity to family and friends		
Availability or quality of a nurse residency program		
Type of hospital: teaching vs. community or private		
"Feel"/support of the work environment		

Activity 14-2: Rocking the Interview

One strategy to land that first exciting position in your top hospital and unit is to shine in the interview. Following are several questions to consider. As you read through the list, consider what to add, and perhaps put a star next to the ones that underscore your most important values and priorities. We have used the HWE standards to frame these as well as Jennifer Hargreaves and Christine Pabico's 2020 article, "How to Choose Your First Nursing Job Wisely." They acknowledge that nurse leaders will carefully interview you to make sure you are the right fit. You should be doing the same interviewing: Is this hospital the right fit for you? Their suggestions come from the American Nurses Credentialing Center Pathway to Excellence Interview Tool (Hargreaves & Pabico, 2020).

Interview Questions to Ask

1. Does your organization use the AACN Standards for an HWE? (Bring a copy to the interview.)
2. Is there Magnet® designation? Beacon units?
3. How long is the nurse residency program? What are the components?
4. Describe the orientation program. Is there a potential to increase it if needed?
5. What are the nurse turnover/retention rate and nurse vacancy rates for the past two years?
6. What do nurses state as their reason for leaving?
7. Are there programs for nursing staff development, such as Crucial Conversations, patient safety, and clinical topics? Are these programs interprofessional, including physicians and other disciplines?

8. Describe the shared governance program and the committees where staff nurses are engaged.
9. What happens when there is conflict or disrespect? Are there policies in place based upon the ANA recommendations?
10. How visible is the nurse manager on the unit? Do they wear scrubs, at least some of the time?
11. What are the biggest challenges nurses face each day? How is the nurse staffing determined? Has there been turnover in the nursing leadership recently?
12. Describe the clinical ladder. Are there awards for nurses? Is the hospital signed on to provide the Daisy Award to nurses?
13. What are the hospital's most notable successes?
14. Describe the programs for nurse well-being.

reflect & journal

- Choosing your first nursing job probably feels stressful, but we hope this chapter has helped you feel a little less so. What are your concerns, fears, and worries about your first job? What elements of your first work environment might alleviate some of those concerns? (Note: Honest sharing from instructor to student to allay fears or mitigate them through an open dialogue is helpful. Perhaps say, "Just like me, you will have choices that reflect your values and ideals.")

- This might be a good time to encourage you to reflect on all the accomplishments you have already achieved, all the challenges you have met with grace and energy, and the many skills you have mastered. Set a timer for 10 minutes and make a list of all you are proud of about yourself. Write quickly, and do not think too much. Just write.

- The importance of "meaningful recognition" came to the fore during the COVID-19 pandemic. Citizens applauded healthcare workers during shift changes. We left our Christmas lights up through the winter to acknowledge their service. Many were celebrated as "heroes." Yet in many hospitals, nurses felt the sting of "unmeaningful recognition," such as free pizzas, buttons, or T-shirts. We often heard nurses say something like, "Don't tell me I'm a hero. Just wear your damn mask." What really is meaningful recognition? Does it depend on the circumstances? On the individual nurse? What meaningful recognition have you received or would you like to receive?

> Consider spending time on the "What Do I Do If I Hate My First Job?" interview that follows this chapter. Ask your students who they will have in their network. They may also want to spend time considering their "dream job" and the influences that may factor into their job decisions (e.g., pressure from parents, etc.).

reference

Hargreaves, J., & Pabico, C. (2020). How to choose your first nursing job wisely. *American Nurse Journal, 15*(5), 30–31.

15
Self-Care for Humanitarian Aid Workers

—Tim Cunningham

what

Read Chapter 15.

- What are the global and humanitarian crises that give rise to the need to deploy healthcare workers?

  - Natural disasters, including floods, earthquakes, tsunamis, and volcanic eruptions
  - Wars, "Global War on Terrorism"

  In addition to refugees, *internally displaced people* are those who are forced to settle in a different, unfamiliar part of their own country or in a camp within their own country. *Asylum seekers* must also flee their country, but because of the situation they will never be able to return. They must seek a new permanent home in another country (Human Rights Watch, 2001). As you can imagine, none of these people, while in flight from their homes, have adequate access to healthcare.

- What are the basic skills needed for nursing work in humanitarian settings?

  - At least two years of nursing experience
  - Language skills
  - Cultural humility
  - Flexibility

- What are the five forms of self-care the author and his colleagues used to care for themselves while helping Ebola victims?

  1. Camaraderie
  2. Music
  3. Humor
  4. Storytelling
  5. Writing

why

Why is self-care even more important for humanitarian aid workers than traditional healthcare workers? What additional stressors do they face?

- Cumbersome, hot, and unforgiving personal protective equipment (PPE)
- Exposure to highly contagious diseases and high mortality rates among healthcare workers
- Shortages of equipment and inadequate technology
- Supply chain challenges ("cold chain")

do

Activity 15-1: Fictional and Nonfictional Healthcare Workers

Read, or reread, a book about healthcare workers in challenging circumstances. We offer a few wonderful choices to get you started. As you read, consider how self-care factors into the subject's work, if at all.

The Plague, by Albert Camus

Cutting for Stone, by Abraham Verghese

The Shift, by Theresa Brown

Being Mortal, by Atul Gawande

Mountains Beyond Mountains, by Tracey Kidder

Activity 15-2: Interview Humanitarian or Pandemic Workers

Interview a student, a nurse peer, or a nursing professor who has worked in a humanitarian setting or during the AIDS epidemic of the 1980s and 1990s. You may also want to interview a nurse who worked during the COVID-19 pandemic. Ask them to describe the work they did and what motivated them to care for their patients. What challenges did they face? How did they take care of themselves? How did they balance their work with the concerns of their families and loved ones?

Activity 15-3: Blogging

We have encouraged you to reflect on your experiences with journal writing, but have you considered sharing your thoughts with others? Many humanitarian workers write online blogs so they can share their experience with others, to feel heard, and with the hope of creating change. Sharing personal narratives can be an opportunity for others, not only humanitarian nurses, to have their voices heard. Consider starting now. As a nursing student or early career nurse, what experiences would be of interest to others? What universal lessons and wisdom are you gaining that you could share with others? Determine your audience and your unique perspective and write a blog post. You might also consider writing an editorial; your school of nursing probably has a communications director who would be willing to help you find a publication "home" for it.

> Depending on the interest among your students, you could do a deeper dive into blogging. This could also be a project for individual students or groups of students during the course:
> - Use resources online or in books about blogging guidelines and tips.
> - Invite your communications director to speak to your class about editorial writing (or blogging if they are experienced in that).
> - Brainstorm with the class their unique points of view and the audiences they could reach. The COVID-19 pandemic has certainly been a time when nursing voices were valuable; unfortunately, few frontline nurses had time to blog. Refer to *Isolation Mask* in Chapter 8 as an example of a nursing voice in the time of COVID. If you have students who would prefer to create poetry, artwork, photography, or music, that would be a powerful way to share the nursing student experience.

reflect & journal

- This chapter reminds us that self-care must be fluid and flexible, not only in humanitarian settings but also in more traditional healthcare environments. When have you been successful in staying flexible during difficult situations? How did that flexibility benefit your well-being?

- Humor has been an important aspect of self-care for this author and others in humanitarian settings. But humor can be dark, and it can diminish those around us. This is especially fraught in healthcare settings. Have you experienced a time when you or others were using humor at other people's expense?

reference

Human Rights Watch. (2001). Refugees, asylum seekers, and internally displaced persons. *Human Rights Watch World Report, 2001.* http://www.hrw.org/wr2k1/

section V
The Heart of a Nurse

16
Mattering: Creating a Rich Work Life

—Julie Haizlip

what

Read Chapter 16.

> This chapter focuses on mattering, a concept that most students will not have considered before. You can help them take the material a step further by inviting them to consider how they will foster their own sense of mattering. Encourage them to be creative, but some ideas include writing a personal mantra; making a scrapbook or memory book of times they have made a difference; or asking a supervisor or patient, "I would like to be helpful to you. What would you like me to do?"

- Mattering is a fascinating concept and one you probably haven't studied before. What are the four domains of interpersonal mattering?

    1. *Awareness* represents the simple idea that others are cognizant of your presence and would miss you if you were not there.

    2. *Importance* to others is their genuine expressed care and concern.

    3. *Reliance* suggests that others depend on you or that your actions affect the lives of those around you.

    4. *Ego-extension* represents the notion that others feel a sense of pride in your successes or disappointment in your failures, as though your performance reflected not only on yourself, but on them.

- Explain the differences between interpersonal mattering and societal mattering.

    > *Interpersonal mattering* entails the domains just mentioned: awareness, importance, reliance, and ego-extension in relation to others; much of this chapter focuses on mattering to peers, colleagues, and supervisors. *Societal mattering* represents one's sense of the value of their work as it contributes to society or meets a societal need.

- In the study conducted by the author, what were the opportunities for nurses to feel like they mattered at work?

    - Experiences with patients
    - Professional expertise
    - Relationships with colleagues
    - Recognition
    - Making a difference

why

- Why is mattering an important concept in the context of nursing education and training? Think not only of "traditional" nursing students, but students who tend to be marginalized.

> Our perceptions of mattering as a person and a student are molded by our senses of fit and belonging in those environments. Flett (2018) states that "going to school is a very different experience for the student who feels like he or she matters compared to the student who feels uncared for and invisible" (p. 225). It is crucial for us to reflect on this sentiment because the psychological environment of the school has a tremendous impact on student learning. Schlossberg (1989) first approached this topic when considering adults who were returning to school. She was concerned that students, especially those who do not fit the norm, who are not made to feel like they belong quickly become marginalized. Her work has inspired educators to consider how best to promote connections for and among students.

- How does a sense of mattering factor into a nurse's sense of well-being and resilience?

> Researchers in the social sciences have linked mattering to a number of essential elements of well-being, such as self-efficacy, personal growth, relatedness, social belonging, and life satisfaction (Flett, 2018; Prilleltensky, 2014; Prilleltensky & Prilleltensky, 2021; Reece et al., 2019). When you feel like you matter, you lead a richer and more connected life.

do

Activity 16-1: When Do I Matter?

Take a moment to think about your experience as a nursing student. Who or what has made you feel like you matter? When have you felt seen or heard? How have you, or could you have, added value? Write or tell the story of a time when you felt like you mattered.

> This can be a powerful classroom activity, using paired interviews. Have students pair off and interview each other about times that they felt as though they mattered to others. Process, or debrief, these interviews as a class, asking interviewees to share stories they heard that touched them. Generate a list of mattering themes. What do the themes have in common?

Activity 16-2: Mattering and Patient Care

Clinicals also provide an opportunity to spend a few extra minutes with a patient. What can you learn about that patient as a person? Perhaps they could share with you what their experience has been with the illness or issue that brought them to the hospital or clinic. How is this experience affecting their life? What do they value most about the care their nurses provide? What advice would they have for you as a future nurse? Asking questions and taking the time to listen to the answers provides a valuable service to anyone but is particularly important if a person is alone, confused, scared, or uncomfortable. You have the potential to make that person feel seen and heard and to show them that they matter. You can add value by helping that individual feel valued. You may also learn something that has been overlooked or not considered by the team caring for that person and can serve everyone involved by bringing that something to light.

Activity 16-3: Do Students Matter?

Clinical instructors and preceptors choose to work with student nurses because they are invested in your education. In addition to learning about physical assessment, medications, and the art of caring for another person, take a moment to learn something about your preceptor. Why did they choose nursing? What do they enjoy most about working with students? What is the most important thing they do in a day's work? Can your preceptor tell you about a time when they felt like they mattered? The answers to these questions will provide you with valuable insight into the profession of nursing and may provide a much-needed boost for your preceptor. We hope you will find that students play an important role in preceptors' sense of mattering.

> Students can interview nursing school faculty, not just clinical preceptors. Students may learn that showing up to class and engaging in discussions and assignments can foster their professor's sense of mattering and well-being. And this will potentially foster their own sense of mattering—they matter to their professors!

reflect & journal

- The chapter ends by pointing out that there will be times you won't receive the feedback or recognition reminding you that you matter. What will you do to foster your own sense of mattering?

- How can you help others feel as if they matter? This can include fellow students, patients, and colleagues.

> Pamela Hobby's essay about her nurse when she was a pediatric cancer patient demonstrates the impact that nurses and care teams have long after the patient leaves the hospital. Ask your students if they have any experience with nurses or doctors that made a difference in their life. They could consider writing a gratitude letter (or mattering letter) to someone who helped them through a difficult time. (They will feel the benefit of writing the letter even if they don't share it with the intended recipient.)

references

Flett, G. L. (2018). *The psychology of mattering: Understanding the human need to be significant.* Academic Press/Elsevier.

Prilleltensky, I. (2014). Meaning-making, mattering and thriving in community psychology: From co-optation to amelioration and transformation. *Psychosocial Intervention, 23*(2), 151–154. https://doi.org/10.1016/j.psi.2014.07.008

Prilleltensky, I., & Prilleltensky, O. (2021). *How people matter: Why it affects health, happiness, love, work, and society.* Cambridge University Press.

Reece, A., Yaden, D., Kellerman, G., Robichaux, A., Goldstein, R., Schwartz, B., Seligman, M., & Baumeister, R. (2019). Mattering is an indicator of organizational health and employee success. *Journal of Positive Psychology, 16*(2), 228–248. https://doi.org/10.1080/17439760.2019.1689416

Schlossberg, N. K. (1989). Marginality and mattering: Key issues in building community. *New Directions for Student Services, 48,* 5–15. https://doi.org/10.1002/ss.37119894803

17
Integrating a Life That Works With a Life That Counts

–Dorrie K. Fontaine

what

Read Chapter 17.

- Describe David Whyte's "three marriages" metaphor.

> A marriage is an intimate close relationship. Many choose a partner to become a spouse or have a long-term committed relationship. This is the first marriage that is typical and understandable. The second marriage is the close relationship most individuals have with their work, often involving a culmination of education and training for a rewarding career. The expression "they are married to their work" may arise from this notion. The third marriage involves delving deeply into the self and your wants, ideals, and values in life. Together the three marriages represent the full spectrum of the life of a nurse.

- List three ways to foster authenticity in your personal and work relationships.

> Bring your true self to work through meaningful conversations and dialogue about the *real* you. Your hobbies, activities outside of work, studies pursued, and family might all be shared in an open way that is true to yourself but does not violate your level of privacy. Connection and belonging can be achieved in the workplace more readily.

- The chapter offers seven specific strategies for creating and maintaining an integrated life. What are they?

    1. Know yourself.
    2. Seek support. Join your professional, specialty organization as one example.
    3. Offer support to others.
    4. Offer gratitude to yourself and others.
    5. Use kindness as your default response.
    6. Develop a spiritual discipline, not in a strict religious sense but in a habit of reflection and deep meaning.
    7. Cultivate a healthy work environment.

why

Why does the author prefer the term "work-life integration" over "work-life balance"?

> Work-life balance can seem an impossibility with the hectic lives of work, home, and sometimes graduate school. Life does not sort into neat boxes, and the concept of integration is a growing one. Work-life integration can lead to synergy among the many roles and a more authentic self. When our lives and roles do not compete with each other, flourishing can occur, as Salzberg (2014) refers to it in *Real Happiness at Work*.

do

Activity 17-1: Pebble in Your Shoe

The author talks about the Joy in Work project that revealed weekend and evening emails were a "pebble in the shoe" of her faculty. To increase joy in the workplace, the school simply stopped weekend and evening emails, as well as the expectation that these off-hours emails must be answered.

Consider a simple change you could make that could greatly improve your happiness and joy. Make that change and see what happens when you no longer have that pebble in your shoe.

Activity 17-2: Eavesdropping

The first step in creating an integrated life is "knowing yourself" so that you will be free and able to reveal yourself to others. Give yourself time and space (at least 30 minutes) to imagine that it's your nursing school graduation celebration. All the most important people in your life are in attendance—family, friends, teachers, colleagues, patients, and more. You notice a group of them talking animatedly, smiling, and nodding. They are talking about how much they love and care about you and why. They share why they admire you, what they value most about you, and how you have had an impact on their lives. You overhear the entire conversation. What do they say?

reflect & journal

- In class, on the job, and at home, do you feel like you can fully be your authentic self? Are you living, studying, or working in a place where you find yourself coding your language or changing your actions to fit certain expectations? What keeps you from being authentic at times? Think about those expectations and their source. Now consider ways you can take steps to either share yourself more fully in these spaces or find spaces that are more supportive of your true self.

- Write a reflection on why you chose to become a nurse. Was it even a choice for you? We're guessing you've probably been asked this question a few times in nursing school, so this time, when you reflect on the "why" about your career choice, write about it in a way that gives you a sense of strength. What did you experience in your life that made you move in the direction of nursing? How did that experience make you better, stronger, and more knowledgeable about the world you live in? As you write, hang onto this journal entry and go back to it when times are tough in nursing school or your career. You can "bounce back" and remember where you came from and use that as a source of strength and resilience.

reference

Salzberg, S. (2014). *Real happiness at work: Meditations for accomplishment, achievement, and peace.* Workman Publishing.

18
Providing Compassionate Care and Addressing Unmet Social Needs Can Reduce Your Burnout

–Sue Hassmiller

what

Read Chapter 18.

- There are two kinds of compassionate care described in this chapter. What do we mean when we talk about "compassionate care"?

> The first is what we typically think of when we consider compassionate care: "sensitivity to suffering in self and others with a commitment to try to alleviate and prevent it" (Gilbert & Choden, 2013). The second is the compassionate care required to address patients' unmet social needs.

- Only 20% of patients' health outcomes are determined by the medical care they receive (University of Wisconsin Population Health Institute, 2014). List at least six nonmedical factors that affect a patient's health.

> - Access to jobs that pay a living wage, safe housing, reliable transportation, walkable neighborhoods, good schools, fresh food, and adequate green spaces (Braveman & Gottlieb, 2014)
> - Good ventilation in their home or apartment
> - Safety in exercising outside
> - Stair-climbing, if falls are a risk
>
> In class, encourage students to generate a list of nonmedical determinants of health.

why

What are the benefits of compassionate care? Why is compassionate care such an important component of self-care?

> The author writes, "But as St. Francis so aptly notes, 'It is in giving that we receive.' The more that you understand about patients and their families and the context in which they live, the more you will be able to care for them, and the more satisfied you will feel. My hope is that you will provide exceptional clinical and compassionate care, including addressing the unmet needs of patients and their families."

do

Activity 18-1: Addressing Unmet Social Needs

Much has been written about *social determinants of health*, or the social factors that have a significant impact on patients' health. These include socioeconomic status, education, neighborhoods, employment, social support, and access to healthcare (Artiga & Hinton, 2018). This chapter describes some of the ways that nurses try to address these needs with food pantries as well as partnerships with social service agencies to connect patients with vital social services. How do your local hospitals identify and address these unmet social needs? How prevalent are these issues in your community? A lot of this information will be available through your local Department of Health and in agencies that address specific needs, such as mental health and substance use disorders and maternal health.

Activity 18-2: Find Your Voice

In the final sidebar, Elizabeth Métraux advises: "You've found your calling, now find your voice—and your people." In this activity, we ask you to inventory your talents and skills that can become your voice as you advocate for your patients. Are you a good speaker? A compelling writer? A natural leader or persuader? When have you used these talents to effect change?

Activity 18-3: Find Your People

Next, find your people. Research advocacy groups at your institution and in your community. What issue are you especially passionate about? What are the national and international organizations that work to address this issue? Finally, learn about the advocacy work done by professional nursing and healthcare groups, such as the American Nurses Association or Partners in Health. Is there an organization that you would like to become a part of?

reflect & journal

- The chapter author shares her personal story of when her husband was in a fatal accident. What behaviors did his nurses, Abby and Kathy, exhibit that made such an impact on her? What impact did Abby and Kathy's compassionate care have on their own well-being?

- Métraux says it is "impossible to separate the well-being of providers from the pain endured by patients." How does it feel to know that your own well-being is woven into the well-being of those around you, especially those who may be suffering deeply? What implications does this have for you?

references

Artiga, S., & Hinton, E. (2018, May). *Beyond health care: The role of social determinants in promoting health and health equity* (Issue Brief). Henry J. Kaiser Family Foundation. https://www.kff.org/disparities-policy/issue-brief/beyond-health-care-the-role-of-social-determinants-in-promoting-health-and-health-equity/

Braveman, P., & Gottlieb, L. (2014). The social determinants of health: It's time to consider the causes of the causes. *Public Health Reports, 129*(1_suppl2), 19–31. https://journals.sagepub.com/doi/abs/10.1177/00333549141291S206

Gilbert, P., & Choden, K. (2013). *Mindful compassion: Using the power of mindfulness and compassion to transform our lives*. Constable-Robinson.

University of Wisconsin Population Health Institute. (2014). *County health rankings key findings*. Robert Wood Johnson Foundation. https://www.countyhealthrankings.org/sites/default/files/2014%20County%20Health%20Rankings%20Key%20Findings.pdf

19
Showing Up With Grit and Grace: How to Lead Under Pressure as a Nurse Leader

–Lili Powell

what

Read Chapter 19.

- How would you define grit? (You may also want to refer to Chapter 2.) How does Manny exhibit grit in this chapter? Provide two examples of grit that you have practiced or witnessed as a nursing student.

> *Grit* can be defined as working passionately and persistently over time toward a goal, or it can be just showing up every day at work determined to do a good job. Manny showed grit by refusing to back down and leave an unhealthy work environment and devising a better way to allow all nurses to get a break. Student examples might be courageously standing up for a colleague or insisting on more staffing in an unsafe situation.

- How would you define grace? How does Manny exhibit grace? List two examples of grace that you have practiced or witnessed as a nursing student.

> *Grace* is thought of as having aspects of kindness, generosity, and compassion for self and others. A sense of calmness under pressure is demonstrated. Manny showed grace when he took on an awareness of the needs of his fellow nurses, not obsessed with just his own needs and wants. But first he had to acknowledge he was not in a "resilient zone" and was depleted and addressed this through healthy eating, sleep, and walking to work for some sunlight. Student comments on seeing grace in others could include their own actions for self-care and what they witnessed team members doing on the unit.

- What does the author mean by the term *leading mindfully*?

> *Leading mindfully* refers to the model Hunter and Powell developed to show how a focus on your internal thoughts and the practice of mindfulness can result in observable actions that are more skillful in the real world to accomplish the work in healthcare. In this way, wise decisions and a calm sense of supporting others happen with intention.

why

Why are grit and grace such important foundations for effective leaders? Please keep in mind that *everyone* is a leader, not just those at the top of the organizational charts.

> Grit and grace are foundational concepts for leading yourself so you can focus on guiding others in the hard work of patient care. Think of the inner and outer work model. Both are needed. Mindfulness practices and focus with intention can help.

As a course instructor, you are aware of your power to determine the effectiveness of your teaching and the "feel" of the classroom. How you show up each day matters. If you are a parent, you know the influence you have on your family's day-to-day well-being simply by how you show up. Encourage your students to recognize the power they have to affect their patients' and colleagues' well-being simply by showing up with grit and grace.

Ask students if they have anyone in their lives who are "peace people." When one of our peace people is in the room, whether it be a friend or colleague, we know that everything is going to be all right. There is something powerful in their presence that can consistently alter situations for the better. Encourage your students to be like Mr. Rogers.

Look for your peace people. What is it about them that makes you feel at peace?

do

Activity 19-1: Resilience Map

Do the same exercise that Manny did, mapping his resilience on a typical day. As you recall, he woke up tired and sluggish, went through stages of hyperarousal during work, crashed and felt irritated and exhausted toward the end of his shift, and came home with no energy left at all. Map your resilience using the example in Figure 19.4. Narrate your map. What do you notice? Are there small changes you can try with the goal of maximizing your time spent in the resilient zone?

Activity 19-2: Wrappers on the Cart

We love that Manny's story epitomizes what so many authors have shared in the textbook, including both the art of reframing and the power of perspective. Manny discovered that he had the capacity to *choose* how he perceived those wrappers on the carts each morning. The circumstance—wrappers on the carts—was always the same, but Manny's thoughts about them changed. Initially he was annoyed and irritated by them. They made him feel unappreciated and put upon. When he changed his thoughts to see the wrappers as reminders that his colleagues, too, were busy and overworked, his thoughts about the wrappers—and his colleagues—changed. He felt compassion toward his coworkers, and one result of this change was Manny's own well-being.

Do you have a pet peeve? What regularly annoys you? Reframe your personal "wrappers on the cart" and see what happens. You have the power to choose.

Activity 19-3: Arrive-Breathe-Connect

Follow the instructions for the Arrive-Breathe-Connect exercise in Chapter 19. For the next week, practice this exercise at least once a day. Which is easier for you to connect to: grit or grace?

reflect & journal

The chapter author writes that "while you perform, you are also leading, because others are consciously and unconsciously picking up on your cues. Whether or not you and others are aware of it, how you show up in the moment leads others through the power of *your* example." We don't always realize how much power we have in any given situation. We have the ability to turn everything around simply by our presence, demeanor, and grace. In the coming week, pay attention to your own power to influence those around you, hopefully in a positive way!

20
Coaching Yourself When Things Are Hard

—McKenzie Harper

what

Read Chapter 20.

- Summarize Adler's four themes of the stories we tell ourselves.

  > **Agency:** When people made sense of their lives with a sense that they were in the driver's seat, as opposed to being batted around at the whims of external forces, they experienced positive trajectories of mental health in the following years.
  >
  > **Communion:** When people described their lives as marked by connections with close others, they experienced positive trends in their mental health in the following years.
  >
  > **Redemption:** When people's stories about difficult or challenging experiences included a shift in the emotional tone towards some positivity, insight, or lesson they drew from the experience, they showed positive trajectories of mental health in the following years.
  >
  > **Contamination:** When people's stories had patterns wherein positive beginnings gave way to negative endings, they showed negative trajectories of mental health in the following years (Adler, 2015).

- What is the purpose of a "tiny narrative"?

  > The challenge is to take something that feels difficult and to ask whether or not it is possible to tell the story of that moment in a way that shared a nugget of wisdom, clarity, or hope without changing the underlying facts of the story (and in under 100 words!).
  >
  > The author acknowledges that there are some life events that cannot be easily framed in this way. Sometimes we need time and distance from difficult situations to gain perspective and to see how they will impact our larger life story. The point is to begin to shape your everyday stories in a way that bends in the direction of the positive and to find the meaning in your experience. It takes time and practice and sometimes outside help to do this.

- List at least two other self-coaching strategies you can use during challenging times.

  > Finding the positive thread
  > Developing a "delight radar" or strengthening our "delight muscle"
  > Practicing gratitude
  > Appreciating the "whole mess"
  > Carefully designed intentions

> Daily practice
> Simple steps
> Just do it (includes facing problems, opening the door and inviting them in to sit on your couch)
> Meditation
> Journaling
> Sticky notes (positive affirmations)

why

The author embraces the phrase "Love Who You Are" in her roles as a teacher and writer. Why might this be the perfect conclusion to your self-care journey using this textbook? (We hope you will continue your journey for years to come!)

> You will face challenges in your nursing career, and your life, and these occurrences are universal in their inevitability. But there are techniques you can use to coach yourself through these difficult times. How you perceive and internalize the events of your life can have a profound impact on your overall well-being. You can coach yourself to "love who you are," especially in those times when you need love the most.

do

Activity 20-1: Write a Tiny Narrative

Be sure to try the tiny narrative exercise that the author shares in this chapter. As a reminder, here are the steps she recommends:

1. Focus on a single small moment—let's try a moment that felt difficult— and think about how it unfolded. Why did this moment matter in your life? Perhaps you sent an email to the wrong person, showed up at a party on the wrong day, or goofed up on a presentation in front of your class. Maybe you scored an "own goal" during a soccer game, but someone comforted you and that person became a good friend. The list of story possibilities is endless!

2. Try writing this story as if you were telling it to a reader with whom you can be completely yourself. Ask yourself how this moment has greater meaning or could offer a message to others. After you write one draft, try editing to limit yourself to about 100 words.

3. Now check in with yourself. Did you first frame your moment as a contamination story or a redemption story? If the former, can you (or did you) reframe it?

4. Uncomfortable with writing? Give it a try! Practice that idea of finding the positive thread, even if it feels hard to grasp.

Activity 20-2: Commit to One Practice for One Week. Start Small.

Try one or more of these strategies. Start small—maybe with the sticky notes and by developing your delight radar. Do *one thing* today. Commit to it for a week.

Meditation

Try a loving-kindness meditation. Here are a few meditation resources:

- Mindful Website: https://www.mindful.org/this-loving-kindness-meditation-is-a-radical-act-of-love
- *Wherever You Go, There You Are,* by Jon Kabat-Zinn
- Tara Brach (https://www.tarabrach.com) is a meditation teacher, psychologist, and author. You can find her guided meditations anywhere that you listen to podcasts.
- Greater Good Science Center: https://ggsc.berkeley.edu

Journaling

Keep a journal. Document your thoughts and emotions when stress arises. This not only helps you identify recurring negative patterns but also provides a tangible outlet for expressing and processing your feelings. You can do this as a note on your phone, too!

Sticky Notes (aka Positive Affirmations)

Develop a repertoire of positive phrases to counteract negative thoughts. When you catch yourself engaging in self-criticism, repeat affirmations like "You are capable," "You got this!" or "You are resilient." Even "You are beautiful" or "You are enough, just as you are." Over time, these affirmations can become powerful tools in changing your self-talk. One strategy is to post these affirmations around your home; who doesn't want to look in the bathroom mirror and see a sticky note that says, "You got this!" each morning? In fact, this would be a great thing to hop up and do right now. If you are living with roommates, they'll appreciate these notes too; your positive affirmations will have a ripple effect. If you'd like to be more private about this project, place your notes in places like your sock drawer, a book you are reading, or on your computer screen.

Go Looking for Joy: Turn on Your Delight Radar

Spend time every day noticing things that bring you joy. These can be tiny things! For example, the way your dog snores while you are working, the way the rain sounds on your roof, a delicious bite of food, or the way a colleague smiles when you walk by.

reflect & journal

The author's message to you—"Love Who You Are"—might be easy to dismiss, but you shouldn't. Find 20 minutes in a quiet place and write all the reasons you love who you are. Are you compassionate, hardworking, or easygoing? What are the qualities that others love and admire about you? Try to stay focused on these gifts that you bring and don't wander off to areas where you think you need improvement. How does it feel to see these qualities written on the page?

Close your eyes and imagine a difficulty that you are having right now. You'll need a mental image for that difficulty (e.g., a dark cloud). Now imagine that you are at home, and you hear a knock at the door. You open the door, and staring you in the face is your difficulty. While your first instinct is to slam the door and lock it, open the door wide and invite that difficulty in. Sit with it on your couch, and ask what you can do to make it feel better. What opportunities for growth and learning exist for you?

references

Adler, J. (2015, May 5). *Our personal stories matter for our mental health*. SPSP. spsp.org/news-center/character-context-blog/our-personal-stories-matter-our-mental-health